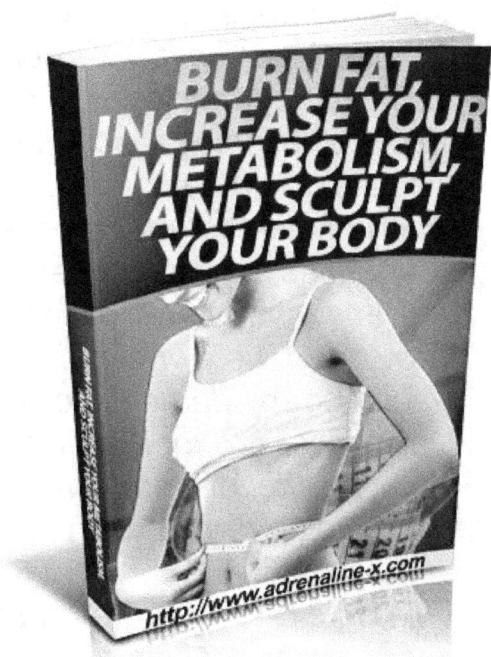

DISCLAIMER: *The information provided by this Web Site or this company is not a substitute for a face-to-face consultation with your physician, and should not be construed as individual medical advice. If a condition persists, please contact your physician. The testimonials on this Web Site are individual cases and do not guarantee that you will get the same results. This site is provided for personal and informational purposes only. This site is not to be construed as any attempt to either prescribe or practice medicine. Neither is the site to be*

Index

Introduction

I know – you've tried everything. Every diet and exercise plan going. At first, everything goes great. You plunge in, full of determination that **this** time it's going to be different.

You might even try a little too hard at first and end up with off-putting aches and pains. Or you may grow impatient with your progress and feel that you're not shaping up quickly enough.

The doubts begin to grow or boredom sets in. Pretty soon you're back right where you started or, worse, you've actually gained a few pounds.

Want to know why? It's because you didn't get your motivation right from the start. You see, every change we make in our lives needs to carefully set up or we end up sabotaging ourselves.

Nowhere is this truer than in the area of diet and fitness. Even top athletes need to adopt the right mindset or they, too, will fail.

But this time, I promise you, things will be different. So long as you follow the steps laid out in this eBook you can and will not only lose excess fat but keep it off – forever!

How? Because we're going to work mind and body together to ensure that you start off motivated and stay motivated. You're going to learn how to get that crucial correct mindset and, what's more, it's going to be FUN.

The human mind and body respond best when they feel safe and relaxed. Push someone out of their comfort zone the wrong way and they will respond by rejecting the whole idea of change.

So, as you work your way through this practical, easy to follow book I want you to enjoy yourself and to understand that you are giving yourself the greatest gift of all: good health.

It doesn't have to be hard and it doesn't have to leave you feeling hungry and miserable. Do it my way and you'll set yourself up for a lifetime of looking and feeling good with absolute ease.

The first thing I'd like you to do is forget everything you ever learned about diet and exercise. That's right – put aside the diet plans and the same old, boring exercise routines and keep an open mind.

At the basis of everything I am about teach you is that your excess weight is simply the result of unhealthy habits you may have learned at an early age or later on in life. The good news is that those habits can be unlearned so that the fat melts away and stays off.

Within this book you will find the kind of nutritional and exercise information that athletes, sports people and dancers use to achieve their perfect, healthy weight. This same information can equally be applied to you. It is suitable for both men and women, young and old, and will yield lasting results.

By applying yourself to my program you will find that the fat not only melts away it stays away. You'll be fitter and happier than you have ever been before.

Why? Because you'll be adopting the same kind of positive mindset that takes an athlete to the top and keeps men and women like you at a healthy weight. It's the kind of thinking that makes it all seem easy and that's because it is.

The wonderful thing about it is that, as you progress, it becomes easier and easier. That's because exercise not only does you good physically, it also has a profound impact on your mental health. You'll be more positive, more productive. You'll look and feel great.

Don't worry – I'm not expecting you to work to Olympic standards but I will promise you world-beating results if you follow this program just as I've outlined it. By following my eating plans and exercises you will finally be fat free forever.

Motivation & Mindset

As you now know, the right mindset is crucial to gaining and maintaining that perfect weight and staying fat free forever. You need to learn and practice techniques that will enable you to stay enthusiastic and focused.

Visualization

One of the best techniques is visualization. Visualization is used by Olympic athletes, top business people and ordinary folk like you and me to mentally rehearse an outcome we desire.

This kind of mental rehearsal is incredibly powerful. By simply picturing the outcome you deeply and passionately desire you can literally make those thoughts come true. The trick, as ever, is to do it the right way.

Visualization works particularly well for fitness as the outcome you desire is so easy to picture. Try it – imagine a slimmer, toned version of yourself.

Now, was that so hard? OK, so it's not quite that simple. There are a number of steps you need to follow in order to achieve optimum results.

I suggest you read these through twice before putting them into action as you will want to relax and run through the necessary steps without having to pause or look back at these notes.

Visualization 1

This first exercise will teach you the basics while simultaneously achieving powerful results. It may seem simple but do not underestimate its effectiveness.

1. Sit comfortably and allow your breathing to slow without forcing it, taking in long, deep breaths and noticing your ribs expand. When you feel calm and relaxed, imagine a large television screen right in front of you. Picture yourself in that screen in bright, vibrant colors.

2. This picture of yourself is as you are now – above your ideal weight. Slowly imagine taking off your outer clothes so you are standing there in your underwear. Focus on your excess weight – go on, be brave and

really examine it. Stare at your bulging belly. Take a good, hard look at your bulging hips and thighs.

3. Take note of your feelings about yourself. What are they? Acceptance? Disgust?

4. Now imagine the entire screen in front of you first of all fading until all the color has left it and then shrinking until it is the size of a postage stamp.

5. Begin to imagine another screen sliding in front of that postage stamp, growing bigger and bigger until it is the size of the old one.

6. Make this new screen even more vibrant and colorful than the last.

7. Imagine yourself in that screen, still in your underwear but now at your ideal weight.

8. How do you feel? Happy? Proud of yourself? Whatever positive feelings

you get, intensify them. Actually feel them in your body. Smile.

9. Now squeeze one hand into a fist to allow your body to retain an imprinted memory of those feelings. Every time you waver in your exercise and nutritional program, repeat that same squeeze and those positive images and feelings will come flooding back to spur you on.

Visualization 2

This one is slightly more advanced and will be especially useful before you start exercising:

1. This time I want you to imagine the screen you created before actually inside your head.

2. Project an image of yourself as you are now on this screen but this time see yourself in your workout clothes.

3. Begin to imagine yourself exercising. Pick out a specific routine from the exercises detailed later on in this eBook. See yourself accomplishing this easily and successfully. ENJOY the exercise! Smile, relax. This is fun. This requires almost no effort. See yourself happy and accomplishing every movement with absolute ease.

4. Now imagine yourself standing tall after the exercise. See the beneficial results. See your stomach already flatter, your muscles leaner and stronger.

5. Repeat with another exercise. This time actually pull your stomach muscles in as you visualize and flex your arms and legs. This again will trigger muscle memory, matching up

the positive images of you exercising and achieving great results with muscular movement.

6. Repeat one more time, each time getting leaner, fitter and stronger.

7. At first, do this before every exercise session. Even when you are well into the program and looking great, repeat this visualization every now and then to stoke up your motivation.

Self-Hypnosis

Self-hypnosis has become immensely popular among exercise professionals and for one very good reason: it works.

So what is self-hypnosis?

Think about all those times you've drifted off into a kind of trance or started to daydream. You may have done it while being totally absorbed in something like a book or a movie. You may even have done it when driving and then wondered how on earth you got to where you were going!

Although this same trance-like state of mind occurs during self-hypnosis the important difference is that you use that state to seed a specific motivation or goal in your brain.

Rather than the popular image of hypnosis as being something like sleep, it is actually a heightened state of awareness. The important thing is that, in this state, you suppress your critical faculties.

Take, for example, your desire to lose weight and keep it off. In your everyday state of mind you might have that thought or desire but that little, critical voice that pops up all too often for most of us will probably start telling you that it's impossible, that you don't deserve this, that you're never going to do it.

Using self-hypnosis means that we can turn that voice off. And once that voice is turned off we can plant positive suggestions much more successfully.

Just imagine how wonderful it must feel to be in a calm, peaceful state where you can convince yourself that anything is possible, that <u>of course</u> you can lose those extra pounds and, what's more, you can stay that way effortlessly.

Sounds good? Then let's do it!

First you have to ask yourself:

What do you want to achieve?

Self-hypnosis works best when you are clear and specific about your goals. It helps to write them down before you start as this can clarify them for you and make them seem more real.

In this case, you need to write down the ideal weight you want to achieve along with the measurements you are aiming to attain. Yes, that means stepping on those scales and getting out that tape measure but that's a good thing. Once you know what you're dealing with, you can set a realistic goal for you.

Once you have written down your goal, you need to:

Write out a plan

You need to plan what you are going to say and the best way to do this is to write yourself a mini script so that you can simply read off it without forgetting anything or stumbling over words.

Repeat your goals

Self hypnosis works best if you write out a number of suggestions for each goal you want to achieve. This will reinforce those suggestions deep into your subconscious in different ways and make it much more likely that your mind will accept the overall goal.

Some people prefer to speak into a digital recorder and then play back the result rather than simply talk themselves into a hypnotic state. This is fine so long as you make sure you keep your language and tone of voice as relevant to you as possible (see 'Personalize it' below for more suggestions). You can, of course, also use the hypnosis mp3s which accompany this eBook.

Create a vision of your success

Find or create some of your own images and symbols to represent and support your goal. Make this real so that they represent precisely how you wish to be. One great way to do this is to make a vision board, finding pictures of slim, healthful people and pasting them on a board so that you can refer to it often and certainly before your self-hypnosis session.

Personalize it

Always use your own words, i.e. the kind of language you would use everyday rather than something you feel you must say. Similarly, use images that appeal and are relevant to your lifestyle so that everything helps support your goal of becoming a better, slimmer you.

Think about suggestions that will really resonate with you. If you particularly hate your fat belly, you could say something like: 'My belly is already slimmer and flatter thanks to my new routine and is going to carry on getting slimmer and flatter.'

Similarly, if you dislike the way you are always out of breath because you are overweight, tell yourself: 'I am now full of life and energy and have all the breath I need. Thanks to my new routine I become more energized every day.'

Use your own voice

If you are going to talk yourself down into a hypnotic state rather than use a recording then start your session in your normal voice and keep it nice and relaxed. Gradually start to slow as your session progresses, softening your voice so that you slip easily into a hypnotic state. Gradually return your voice to normal as you bring yourself out of your hypnotic state and back to reality.

Get comfortable

Always make sure your environment is as calm and peaceful as possible before you begin a self-hypnosis session. Never drive or operate any item of machinery while practicing self-hypnosis. You might like to use props such as soft music or low lighting but, for safety reasons, candles are not recommended.

Relaaaaaax

Start by sitting quietly and focusing internally, allowing your thoughts to just pass through your mind. Don't censor them or worry about anything –

just let everything go and begin to breathe slowly and evenly.

Try, above all, not to judge yourself. You are about to implant new, positive messages in your mind that will enable you to not only reach your weight loss goal but to maintain your fat free self at a healthy weight forever!

Keep breathing and letting go of any anxieties or negativity. Be open to what is about to come and let any distractions simply float away from you.

Count yourself down

Start to imagine that you are descending a long staircase or floating down a stream to help yourself go deeper into a hypnotic state. Begin to count down in your mind at a slow and even pace, slipping into even more profound relaxation. Don't worry if your mind or body at first resists – simply keep counting and you will get there.

Arrive at your own special place

Once you are deeply relaxed, imagine yourself in the perfect environment. This is a place where you feel totally safe and where anything is possible. Make this is as vivid as possible. What can you see, hear and smell?

Once you feel comfortable, imagine yourself in this place only this you is already slimmer and healthier. Begin to implant the suggestions you already planned or simply listen to them if you are using a recording. Allow them to sink in but, again, don't judge or criticize them or yourself in any way.

Set yourself up for next time

Once you have absorbed all those positive, powerful messages include some suggestions to help you when you come out of your trance. You could use something like: 'After this session I will feel twice as motivated and am already looking forward to the next one.'

Count yourself back

At the end of your session, count yourself back to full awareness. Suggest to yourself that when you leave hypnosis you will feel refreshed and alert. Check that you are once again fully awake and alert and enjoy the rest of your day!

Click Here For Self-Hypnosis Audio

Paperback Readers Please Visit URL

http://www.adrenaline-
x.com/download/Self%20Hypnosis.zip

Find Something Better To Do!

Another great technique is what is known as replacement or displacement therapy where you substitute one unhealthy habit with another that is far better for you.

You might immediately think that this is easier said than done. After all, what is nicer than tucking into all that fatty junk food or lounging around as a couch potato?

Many things, actually. And it is those things that might literally save your life. The trick to this technique is to make the new habit far more compelling than the old one and to anchor it in you using some basic NLP.

Now, you may have heard of NLP – Neuro Linguistic Programming – and dismissed it as some kind of manipulative mind-bending stuff. The truth is that, used correctly, it can be a very powerful catalyst for change. See that word 'change'? Did that make you instantly seize up?

The fact is that we humans don't like change. In fact, often we fear it. It's a basic human need to maintain the status quo even if it's slowly killing us. And make no mistake – being overweight will kill you.

Your risk of developing heart disease, cancer, diabetes and a host of other life-threatening conditions is vastly increased if you are obese and heightened if you are even just a little bit overweight.

If that's not enough to convince you then you need to make this more personal. Yes, I agree that death is very personal but you would be surprised how many people shrug and say: 'Gotta go somehow,' and carry on shovelling in that fatty food.

For this exercise, I want you to fill in the columns in the following table. I don't want you to think about your answers too much – just fill them in as they pop into your head. Make sure you fill in each space, even when you think you have run out of ideas. You might be surprised at the results.

Benefits Of Staying As I Am	Benefits Of Getting Slim & Healthy

See any recurring patterns or themes there? See any really **compelling** reasons to stay overweight? Sure, you might think it's nice to eat whatever you like but is it really? Do you really want to keep on filling your body with toxic substances? Or, looking at the second column, can you see why it might be better to make some changes?

There is no right or wrong with this exercise – it is simply designed to set you thinking. Alarm bells should start to ring if you really cannot find any compelling reasons to change and yet you know you are overweight. That's when you really need to make some mental and motivational changes.

If that is the case, I'd like you to go back to the sections on visualization and self-hypnosis and explore why this might be so. You can use visualization to picture yourself getting fatter and sicker and gauge how this feels. Then picture yourself slim, healthy and full of vitality and compare the reactions in yourself.

What feels better? A vibrant, attractive you or the unhealthy version of yourself that you have become? Make no mistake – this is something that you have become. Very few babies are born overweight. Yes, your weight might stem from habits acquired in childhood but it is never too late to change those. All you need is desire mixed with action to achieve fantastic results. And this section is all about creating that desire.

Similarly, you can use self-hypnosis to plant suggestions such as: 'Change does not have to be scary,' or 'I am willing to change my unhealthy habits now.' If you want to carry on these positive affirmations into your waking state then by all means do – they work extremely well.

Once you have gone through these exercises, come back to the table and fill it in again. Have your attitudes changed? By how much? Don't worry if you need to repeat this process a few times. It takes on average 30 days to replace old habits with new ones and somewhat longer to work on our deeper attitudes.

Anchoring

Now that you have produced some compelling reasons why you should lose that weight and keep it off, you can work to anchor those reasons so that they are always there to support your efforts. To do this, find a quiet spot and relax. Take a few deep breaths and begin when you feel calm yet focused.

This bears some similarities to visualization except that the 'anchor' part is where you give yourself a small gesture that you can always repeat to remind your subconscious that your new habits are better than the old ones. So, as with visualization, clear your mind and if any thoughts intrude simply let them go.

Now take one of the reasons why you should get slim and healthy and keep it in mind. Perhaps you wrote something like: 'Having more energy.' So I want you to take yourself back to a time when you were full of energy. Maybe it was when you played a sport you loved or when you were dancing at a great party. If you really cannot think of an occasion then I want you to imagine one, making it as real as possible.

Next, I want you to intensify that thought so that you can really see, feel, hear and smell it. Enjoy it. Enjoy feeling that good. And when that thought is as strong and real as it will ever be, make a small gesture like clenching your fist.

Hold that gesture for a few seconds and then let go. Relax and do something else. You will need to repeat this exercise a few times for it to really become assimilated by your mind and body but you will find it gets easier each time.

Once you have performed this exercise at least three times, I want you to begin to incorporate it into your daily life. Before you begin to exercise, instead of thinking: 'I can't be bothered, I really don't want to do this,' make your gesture and your mind and body will immediately respond.

Using the principle of muscle memory mixed with that subtle subconscious trigger, you will change your attitude to exercise. Literally making yourself remember how good it feels to have all that energy and vitality will spur you on to bring it back into your life or feel more of it.

Anchoring That New Habit

We can also take anchoring a stage further and use it to reinforce activities besides exercise. It's a sad fact that often we overeat out of boredom or unhappiness. Finding something more productive to do can help alleviate both conditions.

Now, that something can be a new hobby or interest. It can be anything from gardening to learning a new language. The important thing here is balance and breaking out of your comfort zone. Yes, this is going to be another change and not something you already do.

Why? Because having the courage to break out of your personal boundaries will boost your confidence enormously. That, in turn, will boost your efforts to get slim and healthy. One breeds the other and it is also important to ensure that boredom is not allowed to set on. So get on out there and find something you've never tried!

Before you attempt whatever it is for the first time, I want you to rehearse it mentally using anchoring. I want you to see yourself easily attaining your new skill and, what is more, enjoying it. To help, you can start by using an image of a time when you did just that – maybe when you mastered riding a bicycle or got an A grade at school.

Just as we did before, I want you to anchor that great feeling using a small gesture. Once you have done that, move on to picturing yourself in your new situation and, again, anchor that. Now when you go to start your new hobby or interest, make that gesture again. You will find that you approach it with exactly the kind of relaxed, confident attitude that breeds success.

At the end of your session, anchor once again and do the same whenever you feel you have made particular progress. This will reinforce your sense of achievement and also deepen your interest in whatever you are doing which, in turn, will ensure that you do not ever again succumb to the sort of boredom that leads to over-eating.

Just as important is that feeling that you are a success at your new hobby. The happier you feel about yourself, the less likely you are to punish yourself by slipping back into unhealthy habits. And believe me, people do this all the time – even those we might consider over-achievers.

Think of the overweight businessman who is materially and professionally a success but, despite this, is unwilling to allow himself the gift of good health. There are, of course, many emotional factors underlying such behaviors but the good news is that almost all of them can be addressed by reinforcing how good we feel about ourselves.

That businessman, deep down, feels a failure in some way and making money is obviously not resolving those feelings. That's because money is an external source of satisfaction and ratification of success. How much better if those feelings come from deep within us.

Many clients of mine report similar self-enrichment when they carry out charity work or engage in an activity such as mentoring. If you go these routes, again I would encourage you to anchor first and to keep on anchoring at intervals until your new habit or interest is firmly integrated in your life.

Adopting an open mindset which embraces rather than fears change is one of the biggest boosters of health and wellbeing that I know. You will find it almost impossible to maintain unhealthy habits if you truly engage in meaningful activity. It simply does not allow you to do yourself this disservice any more.

None of this is going to happen overnight. I would be lying to you if I claimed that. But by setting up the correct mindset as the foundation and cornerstone of your Fat Free Forever program, you are guaranteed success.

In the next sections of this eBook you will find diet and exercise advice that will perfectly complement all this mental work. Except it's not really work, is it? It's fun! What could be better than opening yourself up to a fabulous new you along with a wonderful enriched life?

As you progress through this book, by all means turn back to this section whenever necessary. Play with the exercises and make them your own. This is all about you – a slender, healthy you. I know you can do it. You deserve it.

Fat Free Food

This section is not about food that is totally devoid of fat but rather about the sort of healthy eating that will allow you to become effortlessly slim and stay that way.

Note I said 'eating.' This is not about deprivation or fad diets. This is all about eating right and not depriving yourself of necessary nutrients. You need to equip yourself with the right kind of eating habits so that you maintain a healthy weight. And those eating habits include enjoying food in the right way so that you will simply make the right choices.

Anyone who has ever tried to diet knows that sooner or later you get bored. It's inevitable when your choices are restricted. I therefore want you to look on this section as a re-education rather than a diet. Once you know what and how to eat you will find that the possibilities are endless.

It's also important that you understand that attitude is as important when applied to food as it is to exercise. Too many of us are brought up with or acquire unhealthy notions of what food represents.

We hear and read all kinds of things – that certain foods are 'bad' or 'fattening.' Of course there are foods that contain little if any nutritional value and these are to be avoided but no one food group is inherently bad or fattening provided it is ingested as part of a balanced diet.

Take fat, for example. For many people it's a huge no no. They buy all kinds of low-fat products, unaware that they are actually doing their bodies more harm than good.

Those low-fat products may plaster all kinds of fancy claims on their packaging but read the label closely (and this is something I encourage you always do when shopping) and you will find that what is left out in fat is made up for in increased sugar, salt and chemicals.

As human beings we need fat. It's the densest form of calorific energy we can ingest. The trick is to choose the right kind of fat and that's simple: keep it as natural as possible.

I would rather eat butter any day than the highly processed, hydrogenated polyunsaturated fats prevalent in so many supposedly 'healthy' or 'diet' products. The crucial factor here is that I eat moderate amounts of butter. Rather than slather it on my toast I simply scrape on a small amount.

The same goes for oils. By preference, I'll pick a good olive oil over almost any other both to cook with and to dress salads. You will never find one of those revolting 'diet' dressings in my cupboards because I refuse to feed my body with what is essentially a cocktail of chemicals.

If you don't believe me, read the label. Do you really want to eat a whole bunch of artificial additives and preservatives, some of which may be linked with serious diseases including cancer?

And here's the thing: these additives and preservatives can also cause bloating. So while you are doing your innocent best to slim down, you are actually making yourself look and feel fatter.

The truth is that no natural fat is bad for you provided you follow the 20-40 rule. Keep your fat intake to this percentage of your diet, ensure that it is part of a balanced, healthy eating plan and you will be able to enjoy all kinds of foods while actually losing weight.

Aside from examples such as butter and oil, there are other healthy sources of fat. These include nuts, seeds and avocadoes – all things you may have previously considered to be 'fattening' or unhealthy.

Again, the key is moderation. A handful of Brazil nuts rather than a bowl of salted peanuts, for example. A snack of seeds rather than a low quality chocolate bar full of poor grade hydrogenated fats and sugar.

As for chocolate, that's another thing you can indulge in now and then provided it is at least 70% cocoa solids and the best quality you can afford. This type of chocolate contains less sugar and milk chocolate and will also satisfy your taste buds far more, meaning that you will automatically eat less as you savour it rather than simply gobbling it up.

Fancy a glass of wine? Have it. Just make sure it's a small glass and that you buy organic if at all possible. The same goes for red meat and poultry – eat less of the best you can afford.

Organic, grass-fed beef will be far leaner than the mass produced stuff packed full of hormones. Free range chicken may be more expensive but you will actually receive more for your money as it will not have been injected with water and chemicals to plump it up.

There is strong evidence that the simpler and cleaner we keep our diets the healthier and leaner we become. Another top tip is to only eat what is in season, thereby lessening the chance of your food having been artificially produced and then kept fresh for shipping with quantities of artificial additives.

On the following pages you will find suggestions for healthy sources of fat, carbohydrate and protein. Use these lists in conjunction with the healthy eating sample plans and you will be more than halfway to becoming and remaining fat free forever.

Healthy Sources of Fat

Butter

Olive oil – especially cold-pressed, extra virgin

Sunflower oil

Other unrefined vegetable oils

Fish oil

Nuts

Healthy Sources of Carbohydrate

Fruits	Whole grain cereals
Vegetables	Whole grain pasta
Beans	Some dairy products
Nuts	
Legumes	
Whole grain breads	

Healthy Sources of Protein

Organic, grass-fed red meat	Unrefined dairy products
Free-range chicken	Beans
Duck	Nuts
Goose	Pulses
Fish – preferably not farmed Eggs	
Shellfish	Soy (miso and tempeh)

Keeping The GI Low

As well as choosing healthy foods from the previous tables, you also need to be aware of the Glycemic Index (or GI) of those foods so your choice can be even more informed.

The GI score for each food will tell you the rate at which the sugar in that food will be absorbed. The quicker the GI score, the faster the sugar is absorbed.

The lower the score, the better for you as it will mean sustained, slow release energy that is far less likely to cause stomach bloating or lethargy.

The following tables give the GI values for the popular food groups.

Fruit	GI Score	Carbohydrate	GI Type
Apple	39	12 g	Low G.I
Apple Juice	40	10 g	Low G.I
Apricots	57	7.5 g	Med G.I
Banana	54	23 g	Low-Med G.I
Cantaloupe Melon	65	3 g	Med-High G.I
Cherries	22	10 g	Low G.I
Grapefruit	25	6 g	Low G.I
Grapefruit Juice	48	8 g	Med G.I
Grapes	46	15 g	Low-Med G.I
Kiwi Fruit	52	9 g	Med G.I
Mango	56	14.5 g	Med G.I
Orange	44	6 g	Med G.I
Orange Juice	47	9 g	Med G.I
Peach	42	7 g	Med G.I
Pear	37	10 g	Low G.I
Pineapple	66	10 g	Med-High G.I
Pineapple Juice	46	10 g	Med G.I
Plum	38	9 g	Low G.I
Raisins	64	70 g	Med-High G.I
Strawberries	40	6 g	Low G.I
Sultanas	56	66 g	Med G.I
Watermelon	72	7 g	High G.I
Fruit drink from Concentrate	66	-	High G.I

Fruit Vegetables

Vegetables	GI Score	Carbohydrate	GI Type
Artichoke	15	2 g	Low G.I
Asparagus	14	1.5 g	Low G.I
Bell Peppers	10	2.5 g	Low G.I
Broccoli	10	1.5 g	Low G.I
Brussels Sprouts	16	4 g	Low G.I
Beet	63	8 g	High G.I

Carrot	70	7 g	High G.I
Celery	15	1 g	Low G.I
Cauliflower	15	2.5 g	Low G.I
Cabbage	10	2.5 g	Low G.I
Green Beans	14	3.5 g	Low G.I
Lettuce	10	1.7 g	Low G.I
Mushrooms	10	0.5 g	Low G.I
Onion	10	4 g	Low G.I
Parsnip	98	11 g	High G.I
Potato boiled	56	16.5 g	Med G.I
Potato Mashed	70	16 g	Med G.I
Potato Baked	84	12 g	Med G.I
Potato Sweet	50	20 g	Low-Med G.I
French Fries/Chips (UK)	75	37 g	High G.I
Swede	71	1 g	High G.I
Sweet Corn	55	19 g	Med G.I
Yam	50	32 g	Low-Med G.I

Grains & Pasta

Grain/Pasta	GI Score	Carbohydrate	GI Type
Barley	35	28 g	Low G.I
Buckwheat	55	72 g	Medium G.I
Couscous	65	23 g	Med-High G.I
Cornmeal	70	77 g	High G.I
Rice White Rice	72	30 g	Med-High G.I
Basmati Rice	58	90 g	Medium G.I
Brown Rice	51	31 g	Low-Med G.I
Wheat	48	65 g	Low-Med G.I
Wild Rice	58	21 g	Medium G.I
Rye	35	79 g	Low G.I
Millet	70	24 g	High G.I
Oat Bran	54	11 g	Medium G.I
Pasta regular	49	28 g	Medium G.I
Pasta Gluten free	54	-	Medium G.I
Capellini	46	30 g	Low-Med G.I
Fettuccine	32	29 g	Low G.I
Gnocchi	66	27 g	Med-High G.I
Linguini	52	-	Medium G.I
Instant Noodles	46	13 g	Medium G.I
Rice Noodles	61	25 g	Med-High G.I

Macaroni	45	19 g	Medium G.I
Spaghetti	41	23 g	Low-Med G.I
Barley	35	28 g	Low G.I

Dairy Product	GI Score	Carbohydrate	GI Type
Whole Milk	27	4.5 g (100ml)	Low G.I
Semi-skim Milk	34	5 g (100ml)	Low G.I
Skimmed Milk	32	5 g (100ml)	Low G.I
Goats Milk	-	4.5 g	Low G.I
Chocolate Milk	34	10 g	Low G.I
Instant Non-fat Milk	-	50 g	Low G.I
Evaporated Milk	-	8.5 g	Low G.I
Flavored Soya Milk	30	3.5 g	Low G.I
Sweetened Condensed	-	55 g	Medium G.I
Sweetened Condensed fat-free	-	60 g	Medium G.I
Buttermilk	-	-	Low G.I
Custard	43	17 g	Low-Med G.I
Yogurt natural	35	18 g	Low G.I
Yogurt Low-fat natural	14	7.5 g	Low G.I
Yogurt Low-fat sweetened	33	18 g	Low G.I
Yogurt Low-fat non sweetened	14	10 g	Low G.I
Ice Cream (average)	61	20 g (100g)	Medium G.I
Ice Cream Low-fat	50	24 g	Low-med G.I

Dairy

Breads & Cereals

Bread/Cereal	GI Score	Carbohydrate	GI Type
Bagel	72	65 g	High G.I
Baguette French	95	55 g	Very-High G.I
Bun Hamburger	61	49 g	Med-High G.I
Bread White	71	47 g	High G.I

Bread Wholemeal	69	44 g	High G.I
Bread Gluten free	89	34 g	High G.I
Bread High Fibre	68	45 g	Med-High G.I
Crispbread	81	72 g	High G.I
Croissant	67	38 g	Med-High G.I
Crumpet	69	45 g	High G.I
Donut	76	50 g	High G.I
Linseed Rye Bread	55	31 g	Med G.I
Muffin	44	26 g	Low-Med G.I
Pastry	60	47 g	Med-High G.I
Pita Bread	57	58 g	Med-High G.I
Pizza	60	35 g	Med-High G.I
Rice Cakes	85	78 g	High G.I
Rye Bread	41	14 g	Low-Med G.I
Ryvita	69	55 g	Med-High G.I
Waffles	75	25 g	High G.I

Breakfast Cereals

Breakfast Cereal	GI Score	Carbohydrate	GI Type
All Bran	42	47 g	Low G.I
Cheerios	74	-	High G.I
Coco pops	77	94 g	High G.I

Corn Flakes	84	86 g	High G.I
Muesli	56	70 g	Medium G.I
Oat bran	55	68 g	Medium G.I
Porridge	42	13 g	Low G.I
Rice Krispies	82	90 g	High G.I
Sustain	68	-	Med-High G.I
Sultana Bran	52	68 g	Medium G.I
Shredded Wheat	67	68 g	Med-High G.I
Special K	64	82 g	Med-High G.I
Weetabix	69	76 g	Med-High G.I

Eating Right

To kick start your routine and get you seeing results fast, I recommend a four day plan that will help introduce your body to healthy eating. The reward for this will be a metabolism that is speeded up rather than slowed down by traditional 'diet' plans.

First off, for these initial four days you are going to be eating six small meals a day. It has been proven that such an eating pattern helps initiate weight loss by keeping your metabolism working at a consistently high level.

You will be basing these meals on foods high in healthy monounsaturated fats as well as fruits, vegetables and fiber-rich whole grains, all designed to make sure you feel full.

4 Day Kick-Start

Day One

Breakfast

Small bowl natural probiotic yoghurt mixed with 1 teaspoon honey. Substitute with soy yoghurt if necessary.

1 small pear or apple

3 or 4 Brazil nuts

Herbal tea or unsweetened juice

Lunch

2 slices organic chicken/hard cheese

Small mixed salad scattered with sunflower seeds

Water or herbal tea

Snack smoothie (see recipe)

Dinner

Grilled white fish with handful of mange tout or green beans, 2 or 3 new steamed potatoes drizzled with 1tsp olive oil

Water or herbal tea

Day Two

Breakfast

Small bowl wholegrain, unsweetened cereal with skimmed milk (preferably goat – substitute soy or nut milk as necessary)

4 walnuts

200g melon cubed or sliced

Herbal tea or unsweetened juice

Lunch

Tuna salad made with small tin of tuna in spring water, 2 tbsp natural yoghurt, diced cucumber, tomato and shredded lettuce all mixed together

2 whole-wheat crackers or crispbreads

Water or herbal tea

Snack smoothie (see recipe below)

Dinner

Chicken stroganoff made with small chicken breast, small onion, 1 clove garlic and button mushrooms sautéed in 1tsp olive oil with 1 teaspoon paprika. Stir in two tablespoons natural yoghurt and serve with a handful of cooked brown rice

Water or herbal tea

Day Three

Breakfast

2 slices rye bread toasted and spread thinly with butter and 1 tsp honey

Handful of mixed seeds

1 apple or pear

Herbal tea or unsweetened juice

Lunch

1 bowl vegetable or chicken broth

2 slices hard cheese

2 whole-wheat crackers or crispbreads

Water or herbal tea

Snack smoothie (see recipe below)

Dinner

1 grilled salmon fillet served with mange tout or green beans and 1 small potato thinly sliced and sautéed in 1tsp olive oil

Water or herbal tea

Day Four

Breakfast

1 small bowl of porridge served with skimmed milk and 1 tsp honey if liked. Substitute with wholegrain cereal if you dislike porridge.

1 apple or pear

Herbal tea or unsweetened juice

Lunch

Small bowl of whole-wheat pasta, cooked and then dressed with 1 tbsp olive oil, black pepper and 50g grated hard cheese

1 small mixed salad

1 mango or peach

Water or herbal tea

Snack smoothie (recipe below)

Dinner

1 grilled chicken breast marinated in 1 tsp of soy sauce mixed with 1 tsp honey and served with 1 small, sliced zucchini and 2 or 3 mushrooms sautéed with 1tsp olive oil.

Serve with handful of cooked brown rice

Water or herbal tea

Smoothie Recipes

Apricot, Pineapple & Strawberry Smoothie

1/4 cup crushed pineapple, canned or fresh

1 fresh apricot, diced, seed removed

6 strawberries, frozen

1/2 banana, cut in chunks, frozen

1 1/2 cup water

1 tbsp. skim milk powder

In a blender, process fruit with the rest of the ingredients. Blend until thoroughly mixed and serve.

Banana & Strawberry Smoothie

1 banana, cut in chunks, frozen

6 strawberries, frozen

1 1/4 cup water

1 tbsp. skim milk powder

In a blender, process all the ingredients until thoroughly mixed and serve.

Tropical Smoothie

1/2 mango, peeled, seed removed

1/8 tsp. natural coconut extract

1/2 banana, cut in chunks, frozen

4 strawberries, frozen

6 ice cubes

1 1/4 cups water

In a blender, process all the ingredients until thoroughly mixed and serve.

Banana Berry Smoothie

1/2 banana, cut in chunks, frozen

1/2 pear, cored and sliced

1/4 cup frozen blueberries

1 1/4 cup water

1 tbsp. skim milk powder

1/8 tsp. cinnamon

In a blender, process all the ingredients until thoroughly mixed and serve.

Banana, Orange & Strawberry Smoothie

1/2 banana, cut in chunks, frozen

6 strawberries, frozen

1/2 cup orange juice

1/2 cup water

1 tbsp. skim milk powder

In a blender, process all the ingredients until thoroughly blended and serve.

Banana, Palm Sugar & Apple Smoothie

1 ripe banana, peeled and halved

150 ml natural yoghurt

1 teaspoon palm sugar or honey

1 apple

200 ml skimmed milk or soy milk

In a blender, process all the ingredients until thoroughly blended and serve.

Mango & Orange Smoothie

1 small, ripe mango, peeled and sliced

2 oranges, juiced

Half a lime or lemon, juiced

2 ice cubes

In a blender, process all the ingredients until thoroughly blended and serve.

Peach, Pear & Raspberry Smoothie

1 ripe peach, peeled and sliced

1 ripe pear, peeled, cored and sliced

3 raspberries

2 tbsp yoghurt

1 teaspoon runny honey

2 ice cubes

Put ice and yoghurt in blender and blend for a few seconds until ice is crushed. Still blending, add peach slices then pear. Finally, add raspberries one by one and honey if liked. Blend until smooth.

Rhubarb & Ginger Smoothie

2 stems rhubarb

1 orange

1 teaspoon runny honey

Little grated, fresh ginger

2 ice cubes

Squeeze the juice from the oranges and place in a small pan with the rhubarb, honey, ginger and 1 or 2 tablespoons water. Stir over medium heat until sugar dissolves then cover pan and stew rhubarb over low heat until it softens, adding more water if necessary. Let it cool. Put ice cubes in blender and blend for a few seconds. Add rhubarb mixture and blend until smooth. Drink immediately.

Eating Right – Next Steps

Below you will find suggestions for meal plans suitable for various body types. Remember that these are just suggestions and that you can mix and match sensibly and within reason. If in doubt, refer back to the tables in the previous pages for healthy guidelines.

The following menus are suited to a small to medium sized woman or a small man:

Breakfast	Lunch	Dinner

Small bowl oatmeal with skim milk 1 egg (scrambled or fried) Small glass fresh fruit juice	Tuna Sandwich Mix: 2 oz canned tuna 2 tsp light mayo Serve on 1 slice bread	Fresh Fish Grill: 3 oz fresh fish (salmon, tuna, halibut, etc.) Saute: 11/3 cup zucchini in herbs Serve with: 1 large salad ~1Tbs salad dressing of choice
Breakfast Sandwich 1/2 pita bread 1 egg (scrambled or fried) 1 oz cheese Served with 2 macadamia nuts	Tacos 1 corn tortilla 3 oz seasoned ground meat 1/2 tomato, cubed 1/4 cup onion, chopped Lettuce, chopped Served with Tabasco to taste ~6 chopped olives	Beef Stew Saute: 2/3 tsp olive oil 1/4 cup onion, chopped 1/2 green pepper, chopped ~4 oz (raw weight) beef, cubed Add: 1/2 cup chopped zucchini 1 cup mushrooms 1/4 cup tomato sauce Seasoned with garlic, Worcestershire sauce, salt and pepper

Breakfast	Lunch	Dinner
Small bowl natural, unsweetened yoghurt 1/2 cup grapes	Grilled Chicken Salad 2 oz grilled chicken	Turkey and Greens 2 oz roasted turkey breast Chop and steam:

1 tsp walnuts Spice with vanilla extract and cinnamon or 1 tsp honey	Served over: 2 cup lettuce 1/4 tomato, diced 1/4 cucumber, diced 1/4 green pepper 1/4 cup black beans ~1 Tbs salad dressing of choice	1 1/4 cup kale Saute: 2/3 tsp olive oil, garlic, crushed red peppers, Add steamed kale and mix 1 peach, sliced for dessert
Smoothie Blend together: 1 cup milk 1 cup frozen strawberries Small scoop of cashews	Quesadilla 1 corn tortilla 2 oz cheese 2 Tbs guacamole Jalapenos, sliced Topped with salsa	4 1/2 oz fresh fish, grilled Saute 1 1/3 cup zucchini in herbs Serve with: 1 large salad with 1 1/2 Tbs salad dressing of choice 1 cup fresh strawberries for dessert
Easy Breakfast 1/2 cantaloupe 1/2 cup cottage cheese 6 almonds	Easy Lunch 3 oz deli meat 1 apple 2 macadamia nuts	Easy Chicken Dinner 2 oz baked chicken breast 1 orange 2 macadamia nuts

The following menus are suited to an athletic or larger boned woman or a medium sized man:

Breakfast	Lunch	Dinner
Medium bowl oatmeal with skim milk 1 egg (scrambled or fried) 1 banana Small glass fresh fruit juice	Tuna Sandwich 3 oz canned tuna 3 tsp light mayo 1 slice bread Serve with: 1/2 apple	Fresh Fish 6 oz fresh fish, grilled Saute: 1 1/3 cup zucchini in herbs Serve with: 1 large salad with 2 Tbs salad dressing of choice 2 cups fresh strawberries
Breakfast Sandwich 1/2 pita bread 2 eggs (scrambled or fried) 1 oz cheese 1 oz sliced ham Serve with 1 apple	Deli Sandwich 2 slices of bread 4 1/2 oz sliced deli meat 1 oz cheese 4 Tbs avocado	Beef Stew Saute: 1 1/3 tsp olive oil 1/4 cup onion, chopped 1/2 green pepper, chopped ~8 oz (raw weight) beef, cubed Add: 1 cup zucchini, chopped 1 cup mushrooms,

		chopped 1/2 cup tomato sauce Season with garlic, Worcestershire sauce, salt and pepper Serve with 1 cup fresh strawberries

Breakfast	Lunch	Dinner
Medium bowl natural, unsweetened yoghurt 1/2 cup grapes 1/2 cup strawberries 1 tsp walnuts Spice with vanilla extract and cinnamon or 1 tsp honey	Grilled Chicken Salad 4 oz chicken, grilled 2 cups lettuce 1/4 tomato, chopped 1/4 cucumber, chopped 1/4 green pepper, chopped 1/2 cup black beans 1/4 cup kidney beans ~2 Tbs salad dressing of choice	Turkey and Greens 4 oz turkey breast, roasted 2 1/2 cup kale, chopped and steamed Saute: 1 1/3 tsp olive oil, garlic, crushed red peppers Add kale and mix 2 peaches, sliced for dessert

Easy Breakfast	Easy Lunch	Easy Dinner
1 cantaloupe 1 cup cottage cheese 12 almonds	4 1/2 oz deli meat 1 oz cheese Serve with: 1 apple 1 grapefruit 4 macadamia nuts	4 oz chicken breast, baked 2 oranges 4 macadamia nuts

The following menus are suited to an athletic or larger man:

Breakfast	Lunch	Dinner
Large bowl oatmeal with skim milk 1 egg (scrambled or fried) 1 banana Glass fresh fruit juice	Tuna Sandwich 5 oz tuna, canned 5 tsp light mayo 1 slice bread Serve with 1 1/2 apple	Fresh Fish 7 1/2 oz fresh fish Saute: 1 1/3 cup zucchini in herbs Serve with 1 large salad with 2 1/2 Tbs salad dressing of choice 1/4 cup black beans 2 cups fresh strawberries for dessert
Breakfast Sandwich 1/2 pita bread 2 eggs (scrambled or fried) 2 oz cheese 1 oz ham, sliced Serve with 1 1/2 apple	Deli Sandwich 2 slices bread 4 1/2 oz deli meat 2 oz cheese 5 Tbs avocado 1/2 apple	Fresh Fish 8 1/2 oz fresh fish Saute: 1 1/3 cup zucchini in herbs Serve with 1 large salad with 2 1/2 Tbs salad dressing of choice 1/4 cup black beans

		2 cups fresh strawberries for dessert

Breakfast	Lunch	Dinner
Large bowl natural, unsweetened yoghurt 1/2 cup grapes 1/2 cup strawberries 1 tsp walnuts Spice with vanilla extract and cinnamon or 1 tsp honey	Grilled Chicken Salad 5 oz chicken, grilled 2 cups lettuce 1/4 tomato, chopped 1/4 cucumber, chopped 1/4 green pepper, chopped 1/2 cup black beans 1/2 cup kidney beans 2 1/2 Tbs	Turkey and Greens 5 oz turkey breast, roasted 2 1/2 cup kale, chopped and steamed

Saute: 1 2/3 tsp olive oil, garlic and crushed red peppers Add steamed kale and mix Serve with 3 peaches, sliced |

	salad dressing of choice	
Easy Breakfast 1 1/4 cantaloupe 1 1/4 cup cottage cheese ~ 15 almonds	Easy Lunch 4 1/2 oz deli meat 2 oz cheese 2 1/2 apples 5 macadamia nuts	Easy Dinner 5 oz chicken breast, baked 2 1/2 oranges 5 macadamia nuts

Snacks:

Pick 2 snacks a day from the following list and eat one mid-morning and one mid-afternoon:

1 hard boiled egg
1/2 orange
Sprinkled w/ peanuts

1/2 cup plain yogurt
Sprinkled w/ pecans

1 oz cheese
1/2 apple
1 macadamia nut

1 oz canned chicken or tuna
1 peach
1/2 tsp peanut butter

1 1/2 oz deli-style ham or turkey
1 carrot
5 olives

1 oz mozzarella string cheese
1/2 cup grapes
1 Tbs avocado

1 oz jack cheese
1 Tbs guacamole

1 tomato

1 oz hummus
1/2 tomato
1 1/2 oz feta cheese

1 cup strawberries
1/4 cup cottage cheese
1 macadamia nut

1 poached egg
1/2 slice bread
1/2 tsp peanut butter

1/4 cup cottage cheese
1/2 carrot
3 celery stalks
5 olives

3 oz marinated and baked tofu
1/2 apple
1/2 tsp peanut butter

1 oz tuna
1 large tossed salad
1 tsp salad dressing of choice

1 hard boiled egg
1 large spinach salad
1 tsp oil and vinegar dressing

1 oz grilled turkey breast
1/2 cup blueberries
3 cashews

1/4 cup cottage cheese
1 cup sliced tomato
1/3 tsp olive oil

1 1/2 oz deli-style turkey
1 tangerine
1 Tbs avocado

1 1/2 oz shrimp
2 cups broccoli
6 peanuts

1 1/2 oz feta cheese
1 cup diced tomato
5 olives

1 oz sardines
1/2 nectarine
5 olives

1 oz cheddar cheese melted over
1/2 apple
Sprinkled w/ walnuts

1 1/2 oz scallops
1 sliced cucumber
1/2 tsp tartar sauce

Remember, these eating plans are
guidelines. Follow them for at least two
weeks after your 4 day kick-start program

and then use the healthy recipes in the next section to maintain your new slender frame.

Healthy Recipes

You can mix and match these recipes to maintain your healthy weight.   It is important, however, to stick to the ratio of quantities suggested and not to add unhealthy ingredients such as extra oil or sugar.

Whole-Wheat Spaghetti with Swiss Chard and Pecorino Cheese

Ingredients

1 tablespoon olive oil

2 onions, thinly sliced

2 bunches Swiss chard, trimmed and chopped (about 14 cups)

3 garlic cloves, minced

1 (14 1/2-ounce) can diced tomatoes with juices

1/4 cup dry white wine

1/4 teaspoon dried crushed red pepper
flakes

Salt and pepper

8 ounces whole-wheat spaghetti

1/4 cup pitted kalamata olives, coarsely
chopped

2 tablespoons freshly grated Pecorino
cheese

2 tablespoons toasted pine nuts

Directions

Heat the oil in a heavy large frying pan
over medium heat. Add the onions and
sauté until tender, about 8 minutes. Add
the chard and sauté until it wilts, about 2
minutes. Add the garlic and sauté until
fragrant, about 1 minute. Stir in the
tomatoes with their juices, wine, and red
pepper flakes. Bring to a simmer. Cover
and simmer until the tomatoes begin to
break down and the chard is very tender,
stirring occasionally, about 5 minutes.

Season the chard mixture, to taste, with salt and pepper.

Meanwhile, bring a large pot of salted water to a boil. Add the spaghetti and cook until tender but still firm to the bite, stirring frequently, about 8 to 10 minutes. Drain the spaghetti. Add the spaghetti to the chard mixture and toss to combine. Transfer the pasta to serving bowls. Sprinkle the olives, cheese, and pine nuts and serve.

Serves 4.

Bruschetta with White Beans, Sun-dried Tomatoes and Basil

Ingredients - For the Beans

3/4 cup cannelloni beans

1/4 cup extra-virgin olive oil

1 garlic clove, peeled

1 bay leaf

1/2 teaspoon salt

Ingredients - For the bruschetta and topping

1 small baguette, sliced into thick pieces

1 tablespoon thinly sliced garlic, plus 1 garlic clove, peeled, for coating bread

2 tablespoons extra-virgin olive oil

1/2 teaspoon chili flakes

8 to 10 basil leaves

1/3 cup oil-packed sun-dried tomatoes, drained and sliced

1/4-inch thick

2 tablespoons chopped fresh parsley

Lemon juice

Salt and fresh black pepper

2 ounces ricotta salata cheese, grated

large

Directions

Beans

Rinse the beans well and then put in a 1-quart saucepan. Cover with water to 1-inch over the top of the beans. On medium-high heat, bring to a boil. Immediately take the pot away from the burner, cover and hold for 1 hour. Change the water; add half of the extra-virgin olive oil, 1 garlic clove and the bay leaf. Cook beans on low. Simmer for about 40 minutes or until tender. During last 10 minutes, add 1/2 teaspoon salt. Stir in carefully. Remove from heat and hold in the saucepan with the cooking liquid until cool. This may be done 1 to 2 days before serving, and kept refrigerated.

Bruschetta Topping

Preheat a grill or stove-top grill pan. Grill the bread on both sides until crispy. Be careful on high heat as bread burns easily.

While bread is grilling, in a sauté pan on medium heat, toast the sliced garlic in the olive oil. When it is light golden, add the chili flakes, cook for 10 seconds and then add the basil leaves. Do this carefully, as the basil may spatter some oil.

With a slotted spoon, transfer the beans to the pan. Add 1 to 2 tablespoons of the bean cooking liquid (or liquid from canned beans) and mix all together. Hold warm. Adjust consistency, as necessary, with the bean liquid, a little at a time.

When the basil leaves are wilted, remove mixture from the heat. Add the sun-dried tomatoes and chopped parsley. Toss to combine and adjust the seasoning with lemon juice, to taste, and salt and pepper.

Lightly swipe the remaining garlic clove on 1 side of the bread. Arrange the toasted bruschetta on a serving platter and drizzle with the remaining extra-virgin olive oil. Top each piece with some of the tomato-bean mixture, then evenly divide the ricotta salata over the mixture. Serve warm.

Serves 3.

Three Bean and Beef Chili

Ingredients
1 tablespoon olive oil

1 onion, diced (1 cup)

1 red bell pepper, diced (1 cup)

2 carrots, diced (1/2 cup)

2 teaspoons ground cumin

1 pound extra-lean ground beef (90 percent lean)

1 (28-ounce) can crushed tomatoes

2 cups water

1 chipotle chile in adobo sauce, seeded and minced

2 teaspoons adobo sauce from the can of chipotles

1/2 teaspoon dried oregano

Salt and freshly ground black pepper

1 (15.5-ounce) can black beans, drained and rinsed

1 (15.5-ounce) can kidney beans, drained and rinsed

1 (15.5-ounce) can pinto beans, drained and rinsed

Directions

Heat the oil in large pot or Dutch oven over moderate heat. Add the onion, bell pepper and carrots, cover and cook, stirring occasionally until the vegetables are soft, about 10 minutes. Add the cumin and cook, stirring, for 1 minute. Add the ground beef; raise the heat to high and cook, breaking up the meat with a spoon, until the meat is no longer pink. Stir in the tomatoes, water, chipotle and adobo sauce, oregano and salt and pepper. Cook, partially covered, stirring from time to time, for 30 minutes. Stir in the beans and continue cooking, partially covered, 20 minutes longer. Season, to taste, with salt and pepper.

Serves 8, serving size 1 1/4 cup.

Salmon with Lemon, Capers, and Rosemary

Ingredients

4 (6-ounce) salmon fillets

1/4 cup extra-virgin olive oil

1/2 teaspoon salt

1/2 teaspoon freshly ground black pepper

1 tablespoon minced fresh rosemary leaves

8 lemon slices (about 2 lemons)

1/4 cup lemon juice (about 1 lemon)

1/2 cup Marsala wine (or white wine)

4 teaspoons capers

4 pieces of aluminum foil

Directions

Brush top and bottom of salmon fillets with olive oil and season with salt, pepper, and rosemary. Place each piece of seasoned salmon on a piece of foil large enough to fold over and seal. Top the each piece of salmon with 2 lemon slices, 1 tablespoon of lemon juice, 2 tablespoons of wine, and 1 teaspoon of capers. Wrap up salmon tightly in the foil packets.

Place a grill pan over medium-high heat or preheat a gas or charcoal grill. Place the foil packets on the hot grill and cook for 10 minutes for a 1-inch thick piece of salmon. Serve in the foil packets.
Serves 4.

Chicken Piccata with Pasta and Mushrooms

Ingredients
6 ounces whole-wheat angel hair pasta
1/3 cup all-purpose flour, divided
2 cups reduced-sodium chicken broth
1/2 teaspoon salt, divided
1/4 teaspoon freshly ground pepper
4 chicken cutlets (3/4-1 pound total), trimmed
3 teaspoons extra-virgin olive oil, divided

1 10-ounce package mushrooms, sliced

3 large cloves garlic, minced

1/2 cup white wine

2 tablespoons lemon juice

1/4 cup chopped fresh parsley

2 tablespoons capers, rinsed

2 teaspoons butter

Directions

Bring a large pot of water to a boil. Add pasta and cook until just tender, 4 to 6 minutes or according to package directions. Drain and rinse.

Meanwhile, whisk 5 teaspoons flour and broth in a small bowl until smooth. Place the remaining flour in a shallow dish. Season chicken with 1/4 teaspoon salt and pepper and dredge both sides in the flour. Heat 2 teaspoons oil in a large non-stick skillet over medium heat. Add the chicken and cook until browned and no longer pink in the middle, 2 to 3 minutes per side. Transfer to a plate; keep warm.

Heat the remaining 1 teaspoon oil in the pan over medium-high heat. Add mushrooms and cook, stirring, until they release their juices and begin to brown, about 5 minutes. Transfer to a plate. Add garlic and wine to the pan and cook until reduced by half, 1 to 2 minutes. Stir in the reserved broth-flour mixture, lemon juice and the remaining 1/4 teaspoon salt. Bring to a simmer and cook, stirring, until the sauce is thickened, about 5 minutes.

Stir in parsley, capers, butter and the reserved mushrooms. Measure out 1/2 cup of the mushroom sauce. Toss the pasta in the pan with the remaining sauce. Serve the pasta topped with the chicken and the reserved sauce.

Serves 4.

Chick Pea Salad

Salads made with lots of beans are healthy and full of fiber. This salad can be made with chickpeas, black beans, kidney beans, or black-eyed peas—they're all delicious.

Ingredients
Water for blanching
1 cup broccoli florets
1 15-oz. can chickpeas (garbanzo beans), drained
1 tomato, diced
1 stalk celery, sliced
1/4 cup low fat/fat free mayonnaise or salad dressing
2 Tbsp. lemon juice

1 clove garlic, minced

1 Tbsp. minced fresh parsley

1 Tbsp. chopped onion

Pepper, to taste

Directions

Bring the water to a boil. Add the broccoli and cook for about 2 minutes, then transfer to a colander and immediately run under cold water to stop the cooking process.

In a medium bowl, mix all the ingredients until just combined
Serve over lettuce.

Serves 2 as a meal and 4 as a side dish

Pizza Bianca

Ingredients

Ready made pizza crust

1/8 cup extra-virgin olive oil

5 cloves garlic, minced

1 16 ounce pkg. shredded, reduced fat mozzarella cheese

1/4 cup sliced onion

1/4 cup sliced kalamata olives

1/4 cup quartered canned or bottled artichoke hearts, drained

Pepper, to taste

Directions

Combine the olive oil with the garlic and let sit for about 15 minutes.

Place pizza shell on a pizza pan or baking sheet.

Top with the olive oil and garlic mixture.

Sprinkle the cheese onto the pizza.

Top with the onions, olives, and artichokes.

Bake at 450°F for 10 minutes or until edge of crust is browned and cheese is melted.

Makes 1 pizza

Dulce De Leche Fingers

Ingredients

4 Fajita size soft flour tortillas (34 grams)

4 tablespoons of dulce de leche

1 ounce of sliced almonds

1 large red delicious apple (10 ounces)
sliced and divided in four portions

Directions

Spread 1 tablespoon of dulce de leche on
a flour tortilla.

Sprinkle ¼ ounce of sliced almonds
evenly over the tortilla.

Take ¼ of sliced apple and lay the pieces
2 inches from the edge of the tortilla.

Fold the tortilla covering the sliced apples
and roll.

Repeat with remaining tortillas.

Place tortilla fingers in microwave for 10 seconds.

Serves 4.

Cinnamon Caramel Bananas

Ingredients

4 Bananas

2 tsp Brown sugar

1/2 tsp Vanilla

1/4 tsp Cinnamon

1/2 tablespoon Butter

Vanilla ice cream

Graham crackers

Caramel sauce

Directions

Separate ingredients into 2 bowls.
Slice bananas, top with the rest of the ingredients.

Microwave for about 20-30 seconds, stir. Serve with Ice Cream, crushed up graham crackers and caramel sauce.

Serves 4.

Healthy Cooking Tips

Try this when cooking potatoes: Rather than home fries in butter, layer sliced potatoes (with some onion slices) in a cast iron skillet coated with no stick spray. Brush tops lightly with vegetable oil. Sprinkle with paprika and freshly cracked pepper. Roast the potatoes in the skillet in a 425 degree oven for 20 to 30 minutes or until potatoes are brown on top.

To de-fat homemade broths, soups and stew, prepare the food ahead and chill it. Before reheating the food, lift off the hardened fat formed at the surface. Or, if you don't have the time to chill the food, float a few ice cubes on the surface of the warm liquid to harden the fat. Then remove the fat and discard.

When sautéing onion for flavoring stews, soups and sauces, use non-stick spray, water or stock.

When making a salad dressing, use equal parts water and vinegar and half as much oil. To make up for less intense flavor, add more mustard and herbs.

When making chocolate desserts, use 3 tablespoons of cocoa (if fat is needed to replace the fat in chocolate, add 1 tablespoon or less of vegetable oil) instead of 1 ounce of baking chocolate.

When making cakes and soft-drop cookies, use no more than 2 tablespoons of fat for each cup of flour.

When making muffins, quick breads, or biscuits, use no more than 1-2 tablespoons of fat for each cup of flour.

When making muffins or quick breads, use 3 ripe, very well mashed bananas instead of ½ cup butter or oil.

When baking or cooking, use 3 egg whites and 1 yolk instead of 2 whole eggs; use 2 egg whites instead of 1 whole egg.

When making pie crust, use only ½ cup margarine for every 2 cups of flour.

When you need sour cream, blend 1 cup low fat cottage cheese with 1 tablespoon skim milk and 2 tablespoons lemon juice, substitute plain or nonfat/low fat yogurt, or try some of the reduced fat sour cream substitutes.

Use non-stick vegetable sprays instead of butter.

Use oil instead of shortening, butter, or margarine.

Substitute vegetables or beans for meat, poultry or fish in recipes.

Season your meals with herbs and spices instead of salt.

Lemon juice is also a great low-sodium seasoning.

You can cut the sugar in baked goods down by ¼ or ½, but you cannot do this for cakes or yeast breads.

Read the labels of canned fruits, and look for ones that have been packed in their own juices.

Add vanilla or cinnamon when sugar has been cut to keep foods sweet and interesting.

Replace half of the white flour with whole wheat flour.

Use brown rice instead of white rice.

Add oatmeal or other whole grains to breads.

Add fruits for a sweet treat.

Add more vegetables to your favorite dishes.

Fat Burning Workouts

It is a myth that, in order to burn fat, you need to subject yourself to hours of boring cardio-based exercise. In fact, strength training combined with interval training produces optimum results.

The good news about this is that you can achieve a lot in a short space of time. Even better, you start to see results fast which in turn motivates you to keep going.

A combination of strength and interval training will force your body to burn carbohydrate to supply it with the necessary energy. The right kind of carbohydrate, low GI, is supplied when you follow the nutritional guidelines in this book. Using the exercise and eating tactics in this book synergistically, therefore, will guarantee success.

The following exercises are suitable for all ages and both sexes. If you are pregnant or suffer from any kind of chronic or recurring injury, consult a medical practitioner before beginning any exercise routine. If you feel pain at any time, stop the exercise immediately, rest and seek advice if appropriate. Remember to follow the instructions carefully for a safe, highly effective workout.

Get Your Heart Pumping

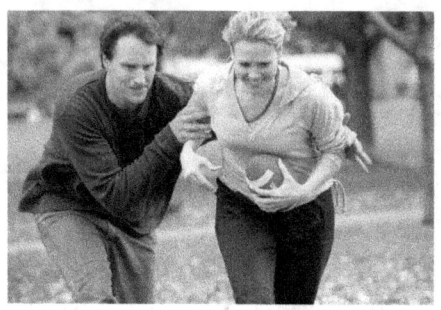

Yes, I know I promised no hours of boring cardio and here I am going to keep my promise. How? By encouraging you to undertake exercise you actually enjoy and to then suggest you reinforce that enjoyment using the NLP techniques such as Anchoring that you learned earlier.

Studies have shown that exercising for at least 30 minutes 5 days a week produces the most beneficial results. The thing is, that exercise can cover a huge range of activities provided that your heart rate is raised to a suitable level for your age and remains at that level for the majority of the exercise period.

Working Out Your Heart Rate

To find your working heart rate, or the optimal level at which you should be exercising, you first need to work out your resting heart rate which will give you a good indication of how your fitness is improving.

The best way to do this is to check your pulse for 60 seconds before you get out of bed in the morning. The fitter you get, the lower this will become.

Working Heart Rate Range Chart
Beats Per Minute (BPM)

Resting Heart Rate	Age							
	30 & Under	31-40	41-45	46-50	51-55	56-60	61-65	Over 65
50-51	140-190	130-190	130-180	120-170	120-170	120-160	110-150	110-150
52-53	140-190	130-190	130-180	120-170	120-170	120-160	110-150	110-150
54-56	140-190	130-190	130-180	120-170	120-170	120-160	110-150	110-150
57-58	140-190	130-190	130-180	130-170	120-170	120-160	110-150	110-150

59-61	140-190	140-190	130-180	130-170	120-170	120-160	110-150	110-150
62-63	140-190	140-190	130-180	130-170	120-170	120-160	120-150	110-150
64-66	140-190	140-190	130-180	130-170	130-170	120-160	120-150	110-150
67-68	140-190	140-190	140-180	130-170	130-170	120-160	120-150	110-150
69-71	150-190	140-190	140-180	130-170	130-170	120-160	120-150	120-150
72-73	150-190	140-190	140-180	130-170	130-170	130-160	120-150	120-150
74-76	150-190	140-190	140-180	130-170	130-170	130-160	120-150	120-150
77-78	150-190	140-190	140-180	130-170	130-170	130-160	120-150	120-150
79-81	150-190	140-190	140-180	130-170	130-170	130-160	120-150	120-150
82-83	150-190	140-190	140-180	140-170	130-170	130-160	120-150	120-150
84-86	150-190	150-190	140-180	140-170	130-170	130-160	120-150	120-150
87-88	150-190	150-190	140-180	140-170	130-170	130-160	130-150	120-150
89-91	150-190	150-190	140-180	140-170	140-170	130-160	130-150	120-150

So What Sort Of Cardio Exercise Should I Do?

This is the fun part – almost anything provided it is safe and follows the criteria for raising your heart rate. I like to mix it up, one day alternating fast walking with jogging in the park, another attending a folk dance class and so on.

The simplest routine is one that is also highly effective – just going for a power walk, arms pumping at sufficient pace will provide a low impact route to stripping excess fat from your body.

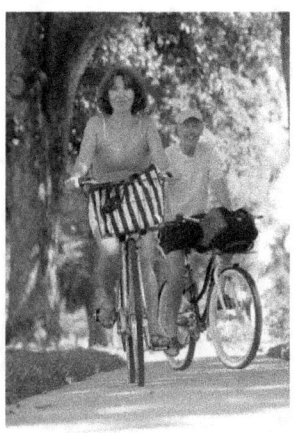

Remember, however, what you learned in the sections on motivation.

It's crucial to keep boredom at bay and to constantly push yourself just that little bit more.

For these reasons, I advocate a class or new hobby that is both physical and fun. Some ideas include:

Tennis

Cycling

Soccer

Volleyball

Hiking

Dancing of all types

Boxing

Canoeing

Rowing

Skiing

Water-skiing

Wind-surfing

Surfing

The possibilities are literally endless and half the joy comes from mastering a new skill which, in turn, boosts your new found confidence.

Ideally, you would split your exercise routine into four or five sessions with one or two devoted to your new hobby or sport and the others mixing up cardio with the routines outlined below.

Of course, there are times when this is not possible due to constraints of work or family, for example, and this is where keeping it simple will also keep you on track.

By this I mean that if you have a basic routine that you can always fall back on you will not fall off the exercise path. Taking a power walk to work/school counts as exercise provided you sustain it for long enough at the right intensity.

Picking out one of the core routines and then performing that for twenty minutes over your lunch break or on your living room carpet will keep up your strength training and your belief that you can do this.

The key is to adapt and to be flexible both in your arrangements and in your attitude. Diets and exercise routines fail when we adopt a defeatist mindset, when we think things like: 'I'm a failure because I didn't go for my run tonight or last night so I might as well slob out on the couch and stuff my face with potato chips.'

The correct attitude would be to think: 'So, I didn't fit in my run tonight. I could always fit in a few exercises before bedtime.' Even a few stretches will keep your body and mind tuned in to the fact that healthy eating and exercise are now simply a non-negotiable part of your life.

With this in mind, I am going to suggest that you mix it up the way I do. To help you keep on track, however, I want you to plan it out each week by filling in the table below. Now, it doesn't matter if you don't stick to the plan absolutely. As I said, stay flexible and substitute one kind of exercise for another. Use your NLP techniques to create and maintain enthusiasm and, above all, enjoy yourself.

To help you, I would suggest planning five days out of seven allowing for two rest days sandwiched between those that involve the most intense activity. As an example, your first week's routine might look something like this:

Monday: Basic Routine
Tuesday: Salsa Class with friend
Wednesday: Rest
Thursday: Lunchtime walk/run for 30 mins with colleague/buddy followed by stretches
Friday: 10 minute jog and straight into Basic Routine
Saturday: Rest
Sunday: Hike with the family

You'll notice that I've scheduled plenty of exercise with either friends or family and that is to help keep my motivation high. We always push ourselves more when we have an exercise buddy or buddies and I would highly encourage you to find someone to exercise with at least part of the time.

Even better, if you follow the Fat Free Forever routine together, working through the book in tandem, then you will find it easier and far more fun to achieve those amazing results. If there is no-one who can exercise with you then don't worry. The pay-off for you is that you will develop iron will-power!

So, with those points in mind, fill in your exercise sheet for week 1. It's a good idea to make a few copies of these sheets and keep them on hand for at least the first four weeks of exercise. That's roughly how long it takes for our bodies to truly absorb and begin to feel the benefit of healthy new habits.

Of course, if you want to plan out each and every week then by all means do and good for you!   Just remember to also schedule in some time for those motivational exercises you learned at the beginning of this book.

The comments section is there for you to record your observations on how your exercise session went. It's here that you can really work on upping your motivation by praising yourself where necessary and by paying close attention to how YOU felt about your session.

Was it fun? Easier than last time? A little more than you expected? Note it all down and, if you keep your exercise sheets together, you'll start to see how you progress over the coming weeks.

You can also use this space to suggest modifications for yourself or even just to write down which particular exercises really worked for you.

Remember, this is all about taking responsibility for your own body and the more you do this the stronger your motivation will be to do the right thing for yourself.

Exercise Sheet	Week:	
Day	**Exercise**	**Comments**
Monday		
Tuesday		
Wednesday		
Thursday		
Friday		
Saturday		
Sunday		

Basic Routine

Perform 3 - 5 days a week for maximum results

You can use this as a complete routine in itself or add it on to the end of a cardio session such as a walk or jog. Performed in its entirety, these will get your heart pumping although probably not at the intensity required to keep your cardiovascular system at peak fitness.

If you like, you can preface this routine with a five or ten minute heart rate raiser such as running on the spot, skipping or simply marching fast, knees high and arms pumping.

You can shorten the routine but it is vital you warm up and cool down properly and perform at least two exercises from each section to ensure that all muscle groups have received balanced attention.

Oh and one more thing – remember to have fun!

Warm-Up

Practice the following exercises slowly while concentrating on your breathing pattern.

BREATHING PREPARATION

Lie on your back on a mat or towel, knees bent, feet hip width apart (measure this from the hip bones, not the outer edge of your hips).

Inhale through the nose, exhale through pursed lips. Upon the exhale draw your navel inward and upward and flatten your tummy. Place one hand on your navel if you like to feel your muscles working.

Draw up the pelvic floor muscles gently. If you don't know where these are, the easiest way of describing them is to say that these are the muscles you use when you are trying to hold in a pee! Continue breathing 5-10 times with these muscles pulled in.

Neck and shoulders should stay loose at all times.

LEG LIFTS

These will stabilise your pelvis and provide a foundation for strong abdominal muscles.

Lie your on back, knees bent, hip distance apart. Inhale to prepare – slowly exhale and lift one knee at a time. Keep fingertips on hip bones to check for movement. Press your lower back into the floor slightly as you lower the legs to avoid arching and over working the back. Keep abdominals pulled up and in. Repeat 5 sets.

ABDOMINAL PREPS

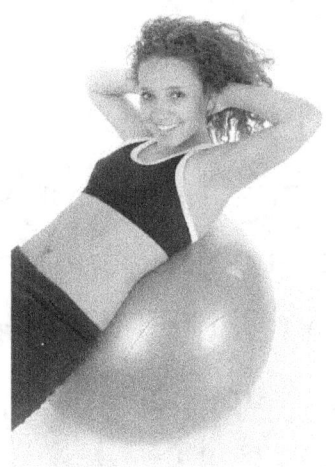

These curls prepare you safely for more challenging abdominal exercises. You can either perform them on the floor or on an exercise ball. One thing to remember:

never jam your chin into your chest, which results in too much compression of the neck.

Lie on your back either on the floor or across an exercise ball, keeping pelvis and spine neutral, which means neither tucking under with your hips nor arching your lower back away from the floor/ball.

Knees are bent, feet hip-width apart on the floor. To prepare, inhale then exhale.

Cradle the back of your neck in your hands, interweaving your fingers. It is VERY IMPORTANT you do not tug on your neck. Gently curl up, pulling in your stomach, aiming to slide your rib cage toward your pelvis.
Hold for a count of two. Slowly lie back down.

Repeat 5-8 times

KNEELING STRETCH

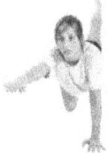

On hands and knees-line up shoulders with hands and knees under hips. Back is straight and neutral. Inhale to prepare – exhale to draw in abdominals, then without shaking or moving torso slowly reach opposite arm and leg.

Hold for 1 full breath, then return.

Repeat 3-4 sets.

GENTLE BACK EXTENSION

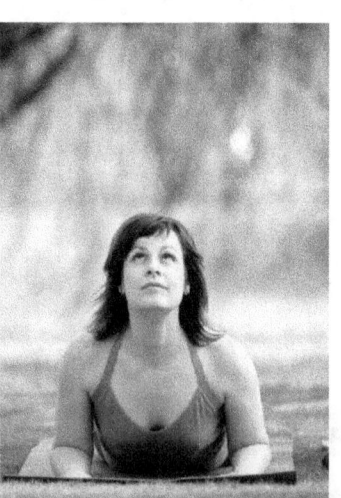

This exercise uses your upper back muscles to lift your head and shoulders off the floor into a gentle back bend instead of pressing up with the arms. Keep your stomach pulled in at all times to protect your lower spine.

Lie on your stomach, keeping pelvis and spine neutral. Legs are straight and together. Elbows are bent, hands by shoulders. To prepare inhale then exhale.

Gently slide shoulder blades down and reach top of head away from tailbone to begin lifting upper back. Allow rib cage to open and maintain bottom ribs in contact with mat.

Hold this position for a count of two and breathe into sides of rib cage without losing your abdominal contraction.

Breathe out and lower upper torso to mat, returning to starting position.

Repeat 5-8 times

REST STRETCH

This exercise stretches your back and abs out the other way, warming up your muscles for the next part of your routine. You can also use it any time to stretch out during your exercise session and it is excellent for general relaxation.

Sit back toward heels, hips lifted, arms wider than shoulders– hold 5 – 10 deep breaths. For tight lower back/hips, place knees wide apart for comfort.

Ideally, you want to be able to rest your rear on your heels and stretch your arms straight out in front of you, hands flat on the floor. If you cannot manage this, then the picture at left shows a safe adaptation.

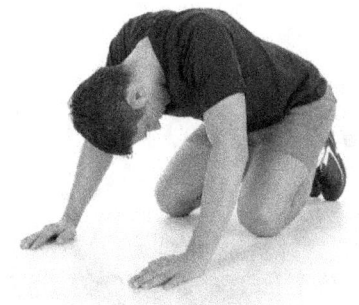

All-Over Workout

Here is the heart of your Basic Routine. Only rest when you absolutely must, so take a short (10-15 sec) rest between two sets of the same exercise.

Before you begin and between this section and the final stretches, find a step or a solid surface on which you can step up that stands around 12 inches from the ground.

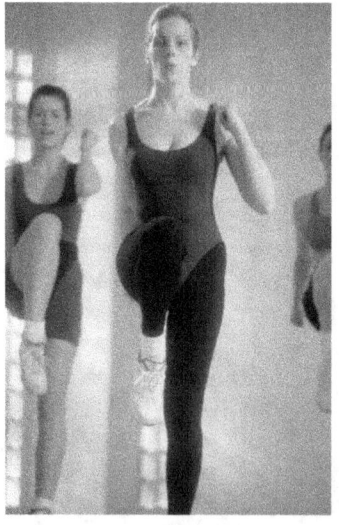

Standing tall and holding in your abdominals, step up and down as fast as you can for 30 seconds. Stop, rest and repeat two more times.

As you get fitter, build this up to one minute, two minutes and so on. The aim is to get you breathing faster than normal but not so fast you cannot carry out a normal conversation while you step.

Tests have proven that this kind of short burst or 'interval' training when combined with other types of exercise yields the best results in obtaining overall fitness and cardiac strength.

Once you have performed your sets, relax and shake out your arms and legs.

Take a 30 seconds rest and then begin the abdominal section that follows.

PILATES CRUNCH

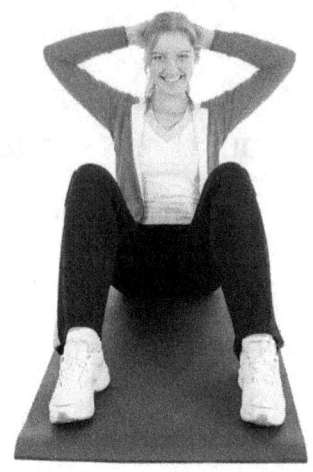

This exercise works your abs with more intensity while remaining safe for your lower back. It is also far more effective than performing hundreds of old-school crunches which tend to develop the neck flexors rather than flatten stomachs as most people cheat and pull up from here rather than using their abdominal muscles.

Start as you did with your abdominal preps, lying on a mat with your knees bent, feet apart and flat on the floor.

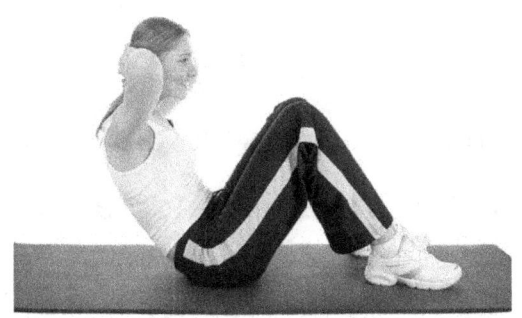

Pull in your abs, navel to spine. Place your hands behind your head and cradle the back of your skull but do not pull on your neck.
`

Still keeping your abs pulled in, slowly curl up, making sure you are not gripping too tightly in your thighs. It's your abdominal muscles that should be working here! Hold for a count of two then slowly lower back. Repeat 5 – 8 times.

ABDOMINAL CURLS WITH LATERAL TWIST

This exercise is designed to tighten your waistline. Start as you did with your abdominal preps, lying on a mat with your knees bent, feet apart and flat on the floor.

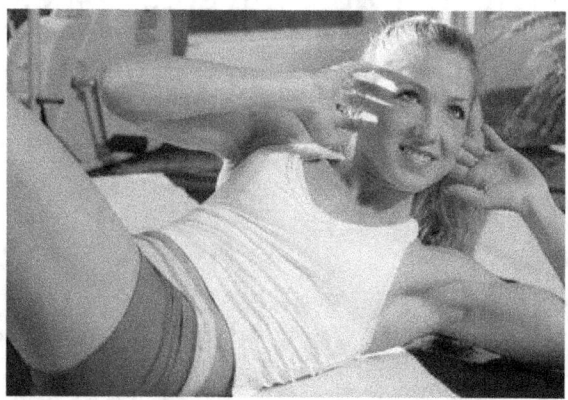

Pull in your abs, navel to spine. Place your hands behind your head and cradle the back of your skull but do not pull on your neck.

If you wish, you can place your hands beside your head as seen here. Still keeping your abs pulled in, slowly curl up, making sure you are not gripping too tightly in your thighs. Don't come up too high but, as you lift your shoulder blades off the floor, begin to twist from the waist towards your opposite hip, keeping your shoulders open.

Return to centre. Repeat on the other side. It is essential that you keep your shoulders open to avoid cheating! You should feel a pull alongside the appropriate side of your waist as you perform this exercise.

Although the actual movement will be very small (your upper torso should move through less than 30 degrees) you should try to go as high as possible. Only your spine should bend, your hips should not move. Do these fairly slowly to avoid using momentum to help.

Perform one on each side before lowering to rest. Perform the entire exercise a total of 8 times. As you become stronger, you can increase the intensity by performing two and then three on each side before lowering to rest.

Repeat 5 – 8 times.

KNEES UP CRUNCH

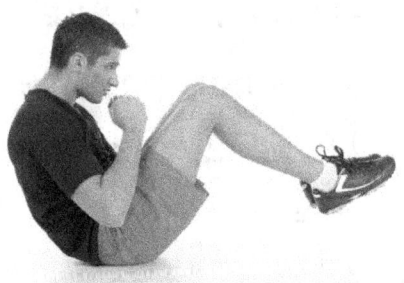

Lie on the floor on your back, knees bent at a 90 degree angle. Raise your legs off the floor until your thighs are perpendicular to your body. Now lift your head and shoulder blades slightly off the floor.

In a curling motion, slowly bring your torso toward your knees.

Hold for two seconds and lower your torso back to the floor, knees at 90 degree angle. Your arms can be crossed in front of your chest, held by your sides as in the picture or rest lightly behind your ears.

CRISS-CROSS

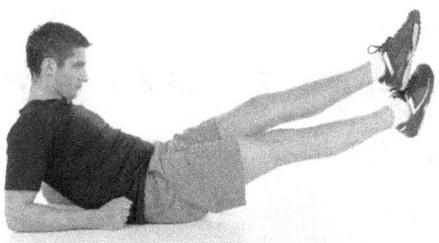

Lie on the floor or a bench, legs stretched out straight. Curl forward from the waist, keeping your legs on the floor for now, and place your hands behind you, palms down, elbows bent, fingers flat or, alternatively, curled into fists as shown here.

Keeping your abdominals pulled in, lean back, bending at the elbows. Raise your legs off the floor to form an angle of around 60 degrees.

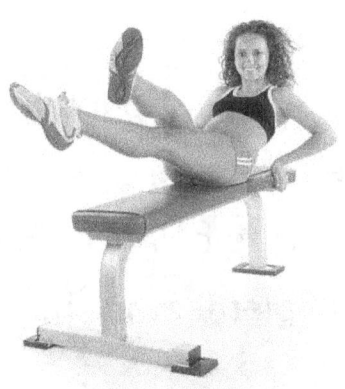

Slowly cross one leg over the other as shown. Reverse and repeat, keeping to a steady rhythm. Criss cross your legs in this way for 20 reps at first, building up so that eventually you can perform 100 with ease.

BRIDGE

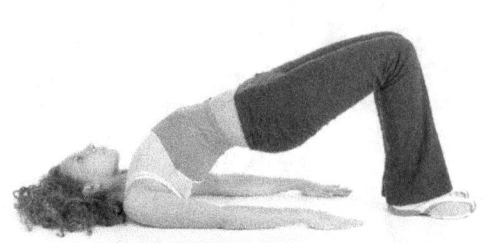

As we've worked your abdominals hard, we need to flex them in the other direction to provide balance and strengthen complementary muscles.

Lie on your back, knees bent, feet hip width apart. Stretch your arms down by your sides, palms down.

Breathe in. On the exhale, pull in your abdominals, tilt your pelvis and roll up through your spine until you are forming the shape above. Keep pushing up through your hips – do not allow them to drop! Also feel that push through your shoulders – this is an excellent strength exercise.

Hold for a count of three.

Breathe in and, on the exhale, slowly lower back through your spine, vertebra by vertebra, keeping your abdominals pulled in all the time. Rest for a count of one. Repeat 5 – 8 times.

PLANK

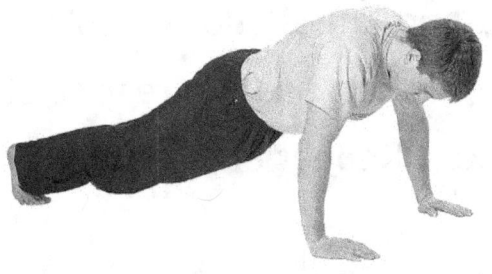

An excellent exercise which will give you all the intensity of crunches in a static pose. This is one of the most effective exercises you can perform for overall core strength and fitness.

You can either do this on the ball or simply using a mat. If on a mat, begin by kneeling on all fours, hands directly under shoulders and knees directly under hips. Extend one leg straight behind you, toes curled under to grip the floor, and then the other. Push your hips up so that you form a straight line. Keep your head in line with your neck and your abs in tight at all times. Hold for a slow count of ten.

Lower yourself back down on to your hands and knees (do not collapse!) and rest. You can use the rest stretch here if you like. Repeat one more time.

As you get stronger, increase the time you hold the position.

PUSH UPS/PRESS UPS

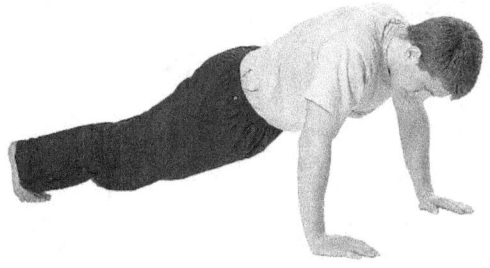

Take up the same position as for plank but this time you are going to lower yourself into a press-up. The important things to remember here are that your hands should be approximately shoulder width apart and that your abdominal muscles should be pulled in at all times.

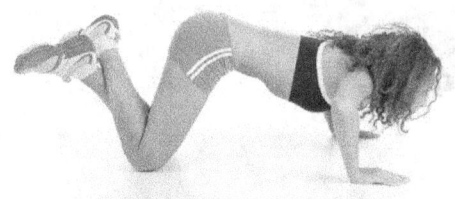

Women may find it easier to perform these with their knees bent as shown but there is no reason why they cannot graduate to a full push up given enough training!

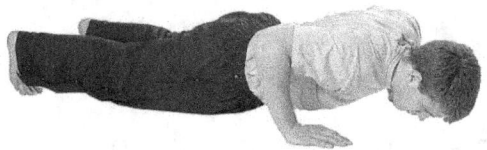

Keeping your head in line with your spine, slowly lower yourself until you are hovering an inch above the floor, making sure that you are taking the strain in both your pectoral (chest) muscles and your arms.

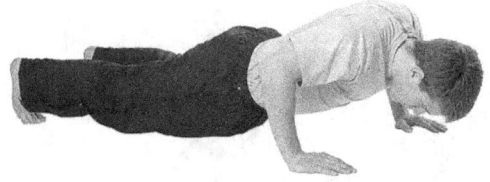

Breathe in and on the out breath push back up to the plank position, straightening your arms but making sure you don't lock them at the elbows.

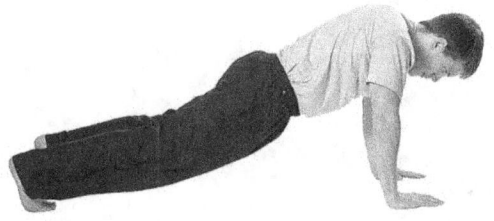

Aim for 10 repetitions but you may find you need to start with 5 and work up. Once you can do 10 with ease, increase your reps until you can perform 3 sets of 20 each time.

RUNNING LUNGES

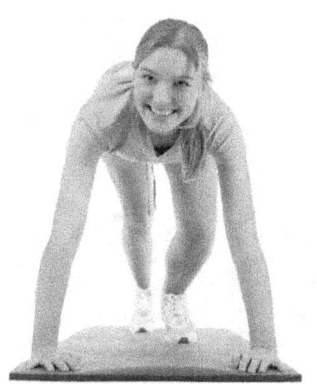

Take up your plank position again but this time you can have your hips slightly raised rather than in line with your spine. This will help your movement to remain natural.

Bring your right leg forward into a lunge position, knee bent, weight on your toes as if you were running and extend your left leg back, curling your toes under for grip. Don't make these movements too big or you will find it more difficult to up the pace.

Swap over so that your left leg is in front and your right leg extended behind you. Build up a rhythm, swapping from leg to leg until it feels like you are running slowly on the spot, aiming to keep it long enough so that you also get the benefit of the lunge.

Build up to 20 reps, 10 on each side. As you get better at this, extend it from 1 to 3 sets per session.

Cool Down

Make sure you do these exercises at the end of every workout so that your muscles have a chance to stretch out. This will lessen the chance of any residual aches the next day and will help keep your morale and motivation high.

DOWNWARD DOG

This yoga-based exercise will ease out your hamstrings and also give your back a good stretch after all that abdominal work.

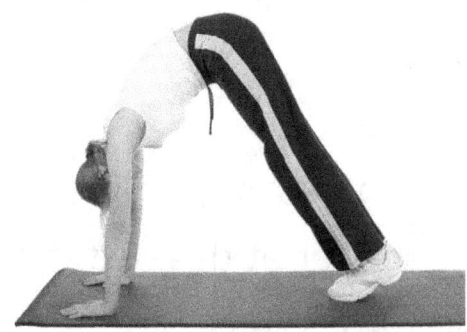

You can either start in plank position or on your hands and knees. Whichever you choose, slowly push back and up until you are in the position shown here.

To increase the stretch, gently push down with your heels and back with your hands so that you feel that you are opening up your armpit area.

Keep your upper back flat and gently try to press in to your spine, imagining it getting even flatter and looser.

Hold this position for 2 or 3 minutes and then either drop down to plank and then to your hands and knees or straight to your hands and knees. Remember to keep your descent slow and graceful – don't just collapse!

Repeat one more time, really enjoying that stretch and feeling the blood flow to your brain, giving you extra energy and thinking power.

SITTING STRETCH

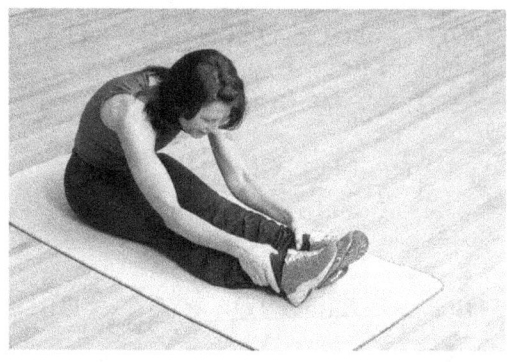

Sit up tall, legs stretched out in front of you, feet and knees together. Slowly bend from the waist and reach forward, aiming to grab hold of your knee, calf or feet – whatever you can manage. Do not force this stretch!

Feel the pull along the back of your legs. Make sure your abdominals are pulled in at all times. Hold for a count of five. Slowly return to sitting upright. Repeat three more times.

INNER LEG STRETCH

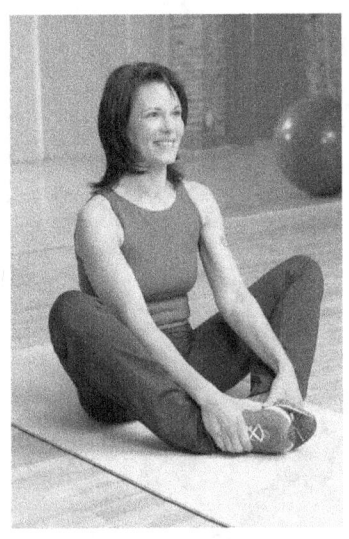

Sit up tall and bend your knees, placing your feet together sole to sole.

Hold your feet and allow your knees to drop out, pulling your abdominals in. Hold for a count of five. Slowly return to the start position. Repeat.

SIDE LUNGE

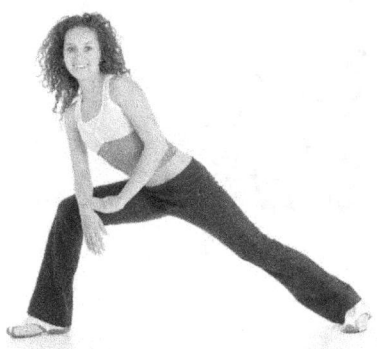

Widen your legs so that you are standing with them about twice hip-width apart.

Bend one knee and lean into that leg, resting your elbow on the leg as shown with the other leg out straight. Hold the position for a count of three. Repeat on the other side, performing three times on each side in total.

SIDE BEND

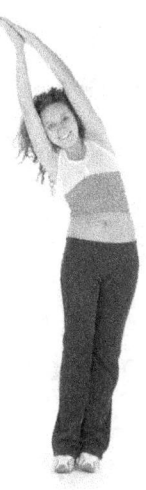

Stand with your back straight and your feet shoulder-width apart.

Place your left hand on your waist and stretch your right arm up above your head, fingertips reaching for the ceiling.

Slowly bend to the right as far as possible.

Use slow, controlled movements and don't jerk. Pause at the top for 1-2 seconds.

Return to the starting position, and then bend to the left. After the set, do a second set.

To increase the intensity, stretch one arm up as before and then the other, either placing palm to palm or clasping the hands together. Bend to the right and then the left, using flow, controlled movements.

STANDING TWIST

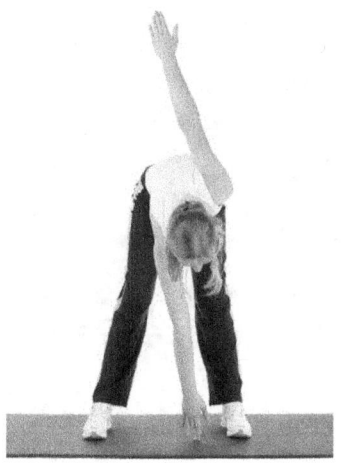

Stand with your feet slightly more than shoulder width apart, arms by your sides.

Bend from the waist, twisting to that you reach opposite hand to foot, aiming to reach beyond the foot.

Return to standing, keeping your abdominals pulled in.

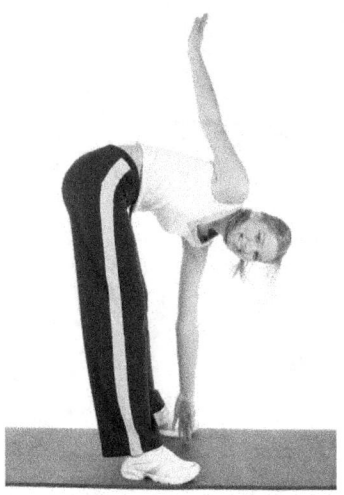

Repeat on the other side. Perform 5 – 10 times.

LAST STRETCH

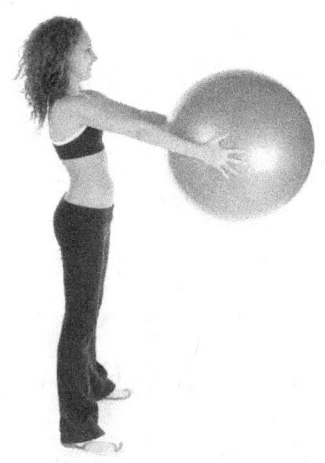

Stand tall, feet hip width apart, shoulders straight but relaxed. Make sure those abs are pulled in!

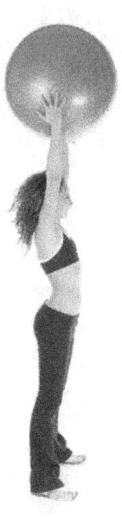

Clasp your hands in front of you loosely and, pulling your abs in even tighter, raise your arms above your head, still clasped together.

Hold for a few seconds and enjoy the stretch. Lower and repeat one more time.

To make this more intense, do it holding a ball between your hands as shown. Don't forget to enjoy the stretch and keep those shoulders loose!

Afterwards, shake out, relax and congratulate yourself on a great workout. Now is a good time to have one of your allotted snacks or a smoothie as you'll keep burning any extra calories for hours.

Click here to access 113 high definition fitness exercises and stretches.

Paperback Readers Please Visit URL

http://www.adrenaline-x.com/fitnessvideos.php

Get Toned Program for Muscle Tone and Cardiovascular Endurance

Disclaimer:

Please recognize the fact that it is your responsibility to work directly with your physician before, during and after seeking information from my site adrenaline-x.com or any other specializing consulting group. As such any

A Warning
The strategy outlined below is Intense.

It's so intense, that you'll have to alter different lifestyle habits aside from work-outs, nutrition and supplementation regiment. Yeah, that's how intense it is to follow. Yet, It's that effective.

This type of plan is not to be used often. I suggest once per year for the duration of 5-8 weeks. Let me make one thing clear though. Let's not confuse intense with dangerous.

If you follow this plan properly, it may even improve your overall health. That's exactly why it is to be used once per year, to boost your health while getting insanely ripped.

What more could you possibly ask for? You're literally getting the best of both worlds.

This plan is designed to give you the best strategy created to make body fat vanish before your eyes. Literally, before your very eyes, in the shortest amount of time possible.

Just to show you exactly what I mean and how fast we are talking, check this out. You will see body fat drop at a rate of .4 - 1% per week following this strategy.

The Get Toned Diet Isn't For Everyone

This can't be said enough; this diet isn't just for the average person.

In fact, if you are closer to 20 % + body fat than you are say to 12-17%, you probably should try out my other products to give you other dietary plans designed to give you a respectable level of body fat year round.

The Formula is simple - weight in lbs x 10cal

Now, does it have to be this way every single day of the week? Not exactly.

The calories you take in will likely change daily, this is unless you eat the same thing over and over again. That wouldn't be any fun would it?

Just in case math isn't a strength, a chart was placed below. Use, it. Remember it.

Bodyweight	Calorie Intake
100 lbs	1000 cal
150 lbs	1500 cal
200 lbs	2000 cal
250 lbs	2500 cal
300 lbs	3000 cal

At this point – a couple of important notes on calories:
1) If you are not seeing any measurable results after the first 7 days, you have 2 things to do.

First, make sure you are sticking to plan exactly how it is written. Not, "well I didn't think eating this would hurt," be strict, more importantly disciplined!

2) If you have been one of those that have been under-eating for long periods of time, your metabolic rate is probably shot to be quite frank. Once you learn proper eating habits and get to a respectable amount of body fat, than please revisit this diet.

The Macronutrient Split:

Alright, you now know the calorie range and the requirements needed before starting this diet, onto the breakdowns!

Protein will make up between 30 and 35% of your daily intake.

Carbs should make up 10 and 15% of your intake. All Carbohydrates should come from vegetable sources. If you can get fresh, that would be ideal.

Fats should make up 50-60% of your intake.

Here is a chart displaying your daily needs:

Bodyweight	CalorieIntake	ProteinIntake	Carb Intake	Fat Intake

100 lbs	1000 cal	75g	25g	66g
150 lbs	1500 cal	113g	38g	100g
200 lbs	2000 cal	150g	50g	132g
250 lbs	2500 cal	188g	63g	167g
300 lbs	3000 cal	226g	76g	200g

Meal Timing:

This part is pretty simple. You will eat four times per day so you will just divide the numbers above by four. This will ensure everything is divided properly and you are eating the right amounts at every single meal. It will seem tedious at first. After a few days, this will be a breeze.

There is another chart below so you get a general idea of what your consumption should be.

Bodyweight	Calorie Intake/Meal	Protein Intake/Meal	Carb Intake/Meal	Fat Intake/Meal
100 lbs	250 cal	19g	7g	17g
150 lbs	375 cal	28g	10g	35g
200 lbs	500 cal	38g	13g	33g
250 lbs	625 cal	47g	16g	42g
300 lbs	750 cal	57g	19g	50g

BCAA & Creatine

These supplements will negate strength and lean mass losses. Basically, you won't feel like crap during this plan.

You'll only feel partially crappy. However, your workouts will stay fun and as productive as possible.

If you tried the Get Ripped Diet Plan without these 2 life saviors, you will see it's like the complete opposite. Seriously, do not skip over these or think it's ok if you don't use them. I like Scivation Extend BCAA and Scitec Ultrapure Creatine 500g. No I do not get paid for saying that either. These are high quality, and fairly cheap.

Here's the protocol:

For those under 199lbs, take 7g of BCAA and 3g of creatine 4x per day for the duration of the Get Ripped Diet. You'll take 1 serving during workouts and 1 serving after workouts. The other 2 you will take in intervals between feeding times.

For those over 199lbs, use 12g of BCAA and 6g of creatine 4x per day for the duration. You'll take 1 serving during workouts and 1 serving after workouts. The other 2 you will take in intervals between feeding times.

In terms of brands, for fat burners I like VPX Sports Meltdown.

Supplement #3
Greens Plus

This has to be one of the best supplements ever to be invented. Seriously, it's that good. This is directly from the product's website.

"Greens Plus is a 100% natural blend of 29 nutrient-rich Superfoods, Sea Vegetables and High-Energy

Herbal Extracts. One serving of Greens Plus delivers more essential vitamins, trace minerals, live enzymes and high-ORAC antioxidants than 5 full servings of fresh fruits and vegetables, and provides every vibrant color in the dietary food spectrum, as recommended by the United States Department of Agriculture."

GREENS Plus® CONTAINS NO yeast, salt, egg, coloring, flavors, irradiation, gluten, preservatives, MSG, corn or dairy products, and NO ADDED sugars, fats or oils.

While on the Get Ripped Diet, Greens Plus will help detoxify your body. This is very important during stages such as rapid fat loss. It helps get rid of the toxins that are being released from your fat cells. It will also help balance out the dietary acids you'll be consuming.

Here's how to use Greens Plus:

Use 1 serving per day, with or without a meal.

Supplement #4

Fish Oil

Do I really have to expound on this one? I didn't think so. Simply take your 7-14g of fish oil per day and you'll be covered.

Supplements #5

Meltdown

Use Meltdown (2 capsules) 2x per day for one week.

I can already hear the cries of expense and the amount of supplements you will be taking. But don't go crazy. Just think for a minute. You won't be spending much money on groceries. Secondly, you won't be on this plan forever, just 1-2 months every 1 to 2 years. So don't think it will be some expense that just goes on and on. It's not, and it won't.

Like I said, all of these supplements these are in place to negate lean muscle mass loss, and to keep you feeling sane during a relatively insane protocol. Sure, you don't have to take these supplements. I'm not going to come to your house and knock on your door. But you better not point fingers when you fall right on your butt, knucklehead!

The Example Meal Plan:

Ok, It's time to get down to the meat and potatoes of the Get Ripped Diet. I made a plan that was quite simply easy to do. Why? Because I'm on the Get Ripped Diet as we speak, so here is my plan:

Wake Up	Breakfast	BCAA/Creatine	Lunch
8oz Water 1 Multi-Vitamin	3 Whole Omega-3 Eggs 2 Pieces of Turkey Bacon 1/2 Cup Green and Red Bell Peppers 28 Grams of Cheddar Cheese 3 Fish Oil Caps 1 Liter Water 2 Meltdown	5 Grams Of BCAA 3 Grams Creatine 1 Liter Water	6 oz 93% Lean Beef (not on a bun) 28 Grams Cheddar Cheese 1 Whole Tomato 1/8 cup Almonds 3 Fish Oil Capsules 2 oz Spinach 1 Liter Water

BCAA/Creatine	Training	Post-Training	Dinner
5 Grams BCAA 3 Grams Creatine 1 Liter Water	5 Grams BCAA 3 Grams Creatine 2 Liters Water	5 Grams BCAA 3 Grams Creatine 1 Liter Water	6 Oz Chicken 28 Grams Feta Cheese 12 Green Olives 1 Whole Tomato 2 Oz Spinach 1 Cup Cucumber 3 Fish Oil Caps 1 Liter Water
Pre-Bed 2 Omega 3 Eggs 30 Grams Cheddar Cheese			

1 Green Bell Pepper 1 Serving Greens + 3 Fish Oil Caps			

Now, remember – This is my plan. Unless you have the same lean mass as I do and you're training as I am, then it would likely work for you. I'm currently 182lbs (4.0% fat) and I workout 5 days a week. My workouts are generally 1.5-2 hours each day.

Some days I may skip a meal and have a serving of BCAA and creatine instead.

Why would I do that? Why not – it helps me get leaner even faster.

Now here's the point of the whole Get Ripped Diet. My plan is always giving me a 0.4%
and 1% body fat loss per week. It's working great, so it's the right plan for me.

The Re-Feed Day:

This is what it's all about. You never thought this day would come, but it's here, the re- feed day. Here's what you do:

-In advance, before you start the plan, pick out these days on a calendar. It will be one day every 12 days. Make sure you mark them down. It will give you some much needed light at the end of the tunnel.

-Until this day arrives, stay disciplined and full steam ahead. No right or left turns into the pizza shop. Be committed and you will have truly earned this day.

-On the 12th day, wake up like it's Thanksgiving. On that day, eat all the stuff you haven't been able to eat while on the Get Ripped Diet.

-Now, hold up, killer. This isn't a license to go buck-wild and act like you just broke outta prison. Don't go too far over 3x your Get Toned Diet calorie guidelines. That means, if you are at 2500 cal per day, you wouldn't go above 7500 cal.

-Lastly, make sure you workout on this day so all these extra calories goes towards building muscle.

People typically gain 4-9 pounds on this day. It's ok - It's normal. It's nothing but glycogen storage and food sitting in your stomach.

Well my friend, you are now armed with some potent information. It's up to you to make use of it...

Hardcore 5 Week Fat Torching Program

If you follow the meal plan and follow the guidelines, you should see results rather quickly. The stricter you are with your following and the longer you remain on the meal plan, the better your results will be. I always tell clients, losing weight is simple...but it's not easy.

You should aim to drink at least a half-gallon of water every day. Don't believe the hype of "diet sodas" and even fruit juice should be limited since it is another source of sugar and therefore empty calories.

ELIMINATE the junk food. No more chips as snacks and no more french fries. Chocolate milk is a perfect post-workout drink as it provides the optimal balance of carbohydrates (sugars) and protein (milk), however, it should not be a part of your daily lunch. No more fried foods. Meats should be baked, broiled, grilled, or pan fried with no more than 1 tablespoon of oil.

Diet

Day 1

Breakfast

3 whole grain waffles

2 tablespoons sugar free syrup

1 cup blueberries

1 cup low fat yogurt

½ cup granola

Lunch

Chicken breast sandwich

3 ounces chicken breast

Whole wheat roll

Vegetables (e.g., lettuce, tomatoes, cucumbers, sprouts, spinach)

Mustard or fat free dressing

1 slice (1 ounce) cheese

1 large apple

1 cup skim milk

Dinner

Taco salad

2 ounces lean ground turkey

½ cup fat free refried beans

Tomatoes and lettuce

½ ounce cheddar cheese

5 small olives

10 tortilla chips

Large banana

1 ounce dark chocolate

Snacks

Pretzels: 50 thin sticks, 2 large twists, or 16 mini twists

1 ounce cheese or 1 cheese stick (string cheese)

1 cup of cut raw veggies (cucumbers, radish, broccoli, cauliflower) and 2 tablespoons of

fat free ranch dip

1 cup of cut watermelon or cantaloupe

Day 2

Breakfast

Egg white omelet w/ mushrooms

1 cup fat free milk

1 banana

Lunch

1 Chef Salad with 4 oz. lean meat

and lots of veggies of your choice

Dinner

10 oz fish

1 cup cooked asparagus

1 cup brown rice

1 cup vegetable soup

Snacks

1 Apple

2 Graham Crackers

Day 3

Breakfast

Turkey bacon

1 medium whole wheat tortilla

2 egg whites and 1 egg

4 tablespoons shredded cheddar cheese

Lunch

Tuna Salad

2 cups salad

2 cups vegetable soup

½ ounce shelled sunflower seeds

2 tablespoons light dressing

1 Banana

Dinner

Chicken stir fry

3 ounces of chicken breast

2 cups of broccoli peas, or green onions

¼ cup teriyaki sauce

½ cup cooked brown rice

1 cup zucchini

1 cup strawberries

Snacks

1 apple, 2 graham crackers

Day 4

Breakfast

Egg white omelet w

spinach, tomato, and   onion

1 cup fat free milk

1 Orange

Lunch

Turkey Burger(No mayo)

Low fat cheese, coleslaw

Chocolate milk

½ cup sliced berries

2 tablespoons almonds

Dinner

Beef and Broccoli Stir Fry

1 cup rice, 1 cup low fat soup.

1 cup green veggies.

Snacks

Crackers: 12 small Wheat Thins or 5 large Triscuits

½ cup of raisins or other dried fruit; 10 walnuts

½ cup low fat cottage cheese

Day 5

Breakfast

Egg white omelet

2 slices turkey bacon

3 small whole grain pancakes

1 cup blueberries

¼ cup of nuts

Lunch

2 cups salad

1 cup soup

2 tablespoons fat free dressing

1 small whole wheat pita

1 small orange

Dinner

10 lean pork (tenderloin)

1 cup brown rice

2 cups low fat soup

2 ounces whole wheat pasta

Sugar free jello

1 apple

Snacks

1 cup yogurt

6 dried apricots

2 ounces beef jerky

Day 6

Breakfast

Protein shake

1 cup milk, 2 scoops whey

protein, 1 cup frozen

Strawberries, ½ banana

Lunch

Stir Fry Vegetables w/ 4 oz. lean meat.

1 cup brown rice

2 slices whole wheat bread

1 cup strawberries

Dinner

5 ounces broiled salmon

1 cup green beans

1 cup cooked rice

1 cup fat free, no sugar added frozen yogurt or ice cream

1 Orange

Snacks

½ cup of applesauce

½ cup of low fat cottage cheese

1 Banana

Day 7

Breakfast

Egg white omelet

3 egg whites and one egg

1 ounce shredded cheddar cheese

2 ounce of lean chopped ham

2 tablespoons ground flaxseed

Chopped vegetables

Lunch

Turkey Burger(No mayo)

Low fat cheese, coleslaw,

Chocolate milk

1 cup watermelon

Dinner

10 oz. fish

1 cup cooked asparagus

1 cup brown rice

1 cup vegetable soup

1 cup cut watermelon

Snacks:

1 ounce of chocolate with 1 fruit

Exercise

Warm Up: Prior to working out you must warm up for 7-10 minutes by performing cardiovascular exercises such as light walking.

Stretching: Stretching exercises are done to prevent injury and help improve performance.

Repeat Day 1 - 5 for 5 weeks with 2 days off a week to rest.

Day 1

Elliptical Machine or Treadmill

5 minutes warm up

level 5 -followed by 8 sets of:

- 60 second's high intensity - level 12

- 90 seconds recovery - level 4-5 -

Then end with a 4 minute cool down

Total of 25-30 minutes

Day 2

Row Machine

1 minute on, 1 minute off, Level 10-15. Row hard for 1 minute, rest for 1 minute.
Repeat this for 10-15 sets.

At a consistent heart rate keep a consistent stroke of 18-22 strokes per minute. Do this for 15-20 minutes.

Day 3

Stationary Bike/Sprinting

Light bike riding for 5 minutes.

After begin your workout as followed

Level 5 50 seconds stationary bike followed by 10 seconds sprint as fast as you can

Level 6 50 seconds stationary bike - 14 seconds sprint

Level 7 40 seconds stationary bike - 14 seconds sprint

Level 8 45 seconds stationary bike - 13 seconds sprint

Level 9 42 seconds stationary bike - 19 seconds sprinting

Level 10 50 seconds stationary bike- 20 seconds sprinting

Level 11 50 seconds stationary bike- 20 seconds sprinting

Level 12 52 seconds stationary bike- 20 seconds sprinting

Level 13 54 seconds stationary bike- 15 seconds sprinting

Level 14 56 seconds stationary bike- 15 seconds sprinting

Level 15 58 seconds stationary bike- 17 seconds sprinting

Level 16 50 seconds stationary bike- 12 seconds sprinting

5 minute cool down with light riding

Day 4

Stair Stepper

Medium speed 5 min warm-up.

40-50 sec. at the highest speed it will go.

30-40 seconds at a low speed to recover.

Repeat 15 to 20 times.

Day 5

Walking – Go for a walk for 30-35

minutes each evening after you have had your dinner. This speeds up the metabolism. You will certainly see results of yourself in 5 weeks flat with this hardcore program.

Conclusion

Fat Free Forever is a program that guarantees you remain trim and healthy so long as you follow the advice given. This means that, if you find yourself giving in to temptation, all you need do is turn back to the sections on mindset and motivation and you'll be right back there on track!

Always remember that you are the one who is in charge of your mind and body. Feed both with the right stuff and you will reap the rewards in the shape of the best body ever and a killer mindset to match.

Keep your eBook and Mp3 files
handy but now it's time to go and
act on all the information you've
received and to try out those
incredible NLP techniques that will
keep you focused on the most
important thing here: YOU.